THE NEUROSCIENCE
OF PSYCHEDELICS

THE NEUROSCIENCE OF PSYCHEDELICS

The Pharmacology of What Makes Us Human

GENÍS ONA, Ph.D.

Park Street Press
Rochester, Vermont

Park Street Press
One Park Street
Rochester, Vermont 05767
www.ParkStPress.com

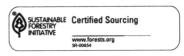

Text stock is SFI certified

Park Street Press is a division of Inner Traditions International

Originally published in 2022 as *Your Brain on Psychedelics* by Argonowta Digital SSL, Madrid, Spain

Note to the Reader: *This book is intended as an informational guide and should not be a substitute for professional medical care or treatment. Neither the author nor the publisher assumes any responsibility for physical, psychological, legal, or social consequences resulting from the ingestion of psychedelic substances or their derivatives.*

Cataloging-in-Publication Data for this title is available from the Library of Congress

ISBN 979-8-88850-004-0 (print)
ISBN 979-8-88850-005-7 (ebook)

Printed and bound in the United States by Lake Book Manufacturing, LLC
The text stock is SFI certified. The Sustainable Forestry Initiative® program promotes sustainable forest management.

10 9 8 7 6 5 4 3 2 1

Text design and layout by Debbie Glogover
This book was typeset in Garamond Premier Pro with Gill Sans MT Pro, Gotham, Nexa, and ITC Legacy Sans used as display fonts

Creative Commons Agreements: Fig. 40 (CC BY 4.0), Fig. 42 (CC BY-SA 3.0), Fig. 43 (CC BY-SA 4.0)

To send correspondence to the author of this book, mail a first-class letter to the author c/o Inner Traditions • Bear & Company, One Park Street, Rochester, VT 05767, and we will forward the communication, or contact the author directly at **genisona.com.**

Scan the QR code and save 25% at InnerTraditions.com. Browse over 2,000 titles on spirituality, the occult, ancient mysteries, new science, holistic health, and natural medicine.

To all subversives, reformers, and agitators.
Your nonconformity and heterodoxy is our hope.

Contents

Foreword

José Carlos Bouso, Ph.D.

Unbounded love. Full acceptance. Absolute understanding. Transformation. Connection. Integrity. Astonishment. Ecstasy. These are some of the most common experiences shared by those who return from a *psychedelic* adventure—which, experienced in moderation, does not seem to leave anyone indifferent. Far from being a contemporary passing fad, after emerging from a few decades of ostracism to which international drug policies had condemned it, the psychedelic experience has been a common practice in the cultural context of humanity, and of radical importance in the cultural construction of the West. The main philosophers of classical Greece participated in the Eleusinian rites, which were celebrated for some two thousand years until the temple of Eleusis, near Athens, was destroyed by Christian fundamentalism, determined from its inception to placate, with force and fierceness if necessary, all spiritual manifestations other than its own. In Eleusis, the ritual involved the drinking of *kykeon*, a hallucinogen whose precise composition has not yet been identified, although recognized experts compare it to modern LSD. It seems that the Eleusinian rites were practiced throughout the entire Greek cultural environment, outside of Greece, and this seems to be attested to by a small chalice found in the area of the ancient city Empuries, a province of Girona, Spain, which was supposedly used to drink the kykeon. We can go back even further, to prehistoric times, and find the case of Selva Pascuala, a Neolithic shelter located in the mountains of Cuenca, Spain. The cave contains a parietal mural in which, according to experts, some psilocybin fungi are depicted, which the primitive inhabitants of the region would use to carry out their explorations of non-ordinary ontological territories.

But the use of psychedelics is not exclusive to the Western cultural tradition. The greatest known diversity of plant hallucinogens is found in South America; in Central America there are also numerous archaeological records of the use of various hallucinogenic plants and mushrooms. There are similar records from Africa and Asia, although with less plant diversity. The anomaly of prosecuting users of hallucinogens (the war on drugs is really a war against those who use them) has been very limited in space (the many countries that are signatories to the International Drug Control Conventions, but not their untamed Indigenous lands) and in time (from 1971 to the present day). Just a few decades in what is surely tens of thousands of years of use. A mere hiccup in the history of humanity.

And it seems that this situation is reversing. On the one hand, in most countries, including for example Spain, only the active ingredients of hallucinogenic plants are controlled, not the plants themselves. And in countries where the plants are controlled, like the United States, a social movement is emerging that calls for decriminalization, something that has already been adopted, in fact, in some states and that, as happened with marijuana before, is producing a chain reaction spreading to other states. Psilocybin mushrooms are already sold in stores in Canada, and the government has authorized the compassionate use of hallucinogens (for patients who have had other treatments fail). For the rest of the planet, ceremonies with ayahuasca, psilocybin mushrooms, or peyote are in the process of global expansion (with their pros and cons, like everything else). Cheap and homemade cultivation methods are easily accessible to everyone, and the array of noncontrolled substances available in informal trafficking networks (thanks to prohibition, which has sharpened the ingenuity of society, new drugs were created when the old ones started being controlled) is the largest in the entire history of mankind. So on that front, although there are still occasional arrests and persecutions, things have gotten so out of hand that, in reality, there is no turning back. What will happen in this race ahead remains to be seen, for at least in the case of ayahuasca, peyote, and iboga, plant resources are limited and may not be enough to supply all the people interested in them. It is an element worth reflecting upon.

On the other hand, we find that the active ingredients controlled in the most restrictive lists, such as LSD, psilocybin, mescaline, DMT, or MDMA, to give the most notorious examples, are becoming the subject of scientific research. Some of them, such as psilocybin for the treatment of depression, or MDMA for post-traumatic stress disorder (PTSD), are in such advanced stages of development that they are expected to be available for clinical use by 2023/24. We will then find ourselves in the paradox that for the same substance one can grow at home or buy on the deep web at absurdly low prices, one will have to pay a fortune for a psychiatrist to administer it. We are already seeing this in the case of ketamine for the treatment of depression. A vial of ketamine or S-ketamine (the racemic one that is also used in clinics) costs just two euros, and contains several dozen therapeutic doses. Its equivalent as an authorized medication for depression costs about five thousand euros, containing the same active ingredient, with a different pharmaceutical preparation, and a much higher price. For this reason, the majority of ketamine treatment centers, at least in Spain, continue to use "run of the mill" ketamine, for obvious reasons. A third option is beginning to emerge in the case of easily accessible drugs, such as MDMA, psilocybin, or ketamine itself: centers are allowing patients to bring the substance, purchased by themselves, and taking it at the consultation under medical supervision.

It will be interesting to see how all these tensions are resolved: on the one hand, as has already been said, the globalization of ceremonies with traditional plants; on the other, the medicalization of controlled hallucinogens and, finally, a possible use of the same active ingredients that are authorized but obtained on the illicit market because of their lower price. In a rational world, we would expect these tensions to be resolved rationally, generating as many possibilities as needed, and where the safety of patients or participants in ceremonies takes precedence. However, in the irrational world we live in, irrational possibilities may include groups asking for the criminal prosecution of other groups; corporatism establishing itself as dominant over other groups (whichever group has the authority to decide the fate of other groups); sensationalism in the media attacking certain ways of doing things and recognizing other ways as the only legitimate ones; and politicians incapable of understanding the complexity of these problems, forcefully applying simple solutions to complex issues, thus generating more harm than good. In short, nothing that we do not already know, having seen the management of similar problems in Spain, for example, from the legalization of cannabis for medical use to the management of the COVID-19 pandemic. Whatever the future holds, its impact will of course be fascinating in the social field. It remains to be seen whether the political and administrative realms will be up to the task and how many victims there will be before that happens, if and when it happens.

That is why a book like this is so pertinent now. It does not deal with social issues, but rather brings us up to date on the current scientific knowledge of the functioning of all these substances, for which so many names have been sought, without consensus. In this book about such an arduous discipline as pharmacology, the young psychologist and pharmacologist Genís Ona makes an informative, entertaining, and, as far as the subject allows, understandable approach to the pharmacology, psychopharmacology, and neuropharmacology of hallucinogens. To understand the pharmacology of hallucinogens is to understand the essence of what makes us human: beings capable of experiencing those ineffable sensations with which this foreword began. Hallucinogens allow us to access unusual spaces of reality, thus becoming a source of knowledge, not of psychopathology. This is how they have been used since time immemorial, and this is also the most

interesting way of contemporary use. It is still paradoxical that when
the therapeutic value of hallucinogens is recognized (once their safety
and efficacy as drugs to treat mental health problems have been demonstrated), what is being implicitly recognized is the therapeutic value
of hallucinations. And, perhaps, parallel to this, a less pathological
view of some human psychological experiences that are currently considered diseases will begin to emerge, despite the lack of evidence on
their physiopathogenesis.

In this sense, Genís Ona also wonderfully guides us along the
path of pharmacological research and its direction—how, in the years
when psychedelics were considered psychopathology-inducing substances, the mechanisms by which they produced aberrant psychological effects were sought in their neuropharmacology (the interest
back then being the cause of diseases such as schizophrenia). Today
the outlook is quite different and we find studies where hallucinogens have been shown to improve prosocial behavior or counteract the
neurobiological mechanisms of anxiety. So we have gone from looking
for the bases of human psychopathology to exploring the bases of its
healing mechanisms. The curious thing about the matter is that the
mechanisms are the same and what varies is the way in which they
are viewed. Before, they were viewed as the mechanisms by which our
brain developed schizophrenia and today they are viewed as the ones
that can cure depression. The scientific investigation of hallucinogens
is the best example of how science is not as objective as some claim it
to be but is as imbricated in social context as any other human activity. Social context will decide what hallucinogens are useful for, and
that is what will guide their pharmacological research, yielding better
insight into their neurobiological bases.

But why a book on the pharmacology of hallucinogens? What is
so interesting about pharmacology to dedicate a popular science book
to it? Beyond what the author already comments in his introduction,
that is, that although we do not talk about the mechanism of action
of drugs in our everyday lives, medicines are in fact part of that daily
life, and it never hurts to know something about what they do to our

body (and what our body does with medicines). In the case of hallucinogenic drugs, the interest, in my opinion, is enormous. We are talking about substances with a minimal effect on the body that induce a maximum state of consciousness. Hallucinogenic drugs are that link between the extremely material (our body) and the extremely spiritual (our conscience absolutely exposed). In a way, hallucinogens are a kind of philosophers' stone that, when in contact with a series of brain receptors, produces an amazing transformation of reality, in which, on the subjective plane, the spiritual is separated from the physical. The subjective experience with hallucinogens is therefore extremely spiritual: in its peak effect, the body disappears and only the spirit remains, at the mercy of transformation, in its most radical essence—a sentient, knowing, and understanding spirit. For Indigenous cultures, hallucinogens are the vehicle to enter a spiritual territory that is as real, if not more so, than reality itself, from which rise myths, cosmogonies, and the knowledge of the origins of disease and its sources for correction, where the shamans carry out their medical acts. Their concepts of health and disease have nothing to do with ours. And, Westerners being so spiritually illiterate, these substances allow us to access understandings about the nature of reality that can later serve us in our daily lives, as much therapeutically as ontologically and transcendentally (one of the uses of psychedelics being recovered is precisely in patients with terminal illnesses, preparing them to face death). If this is so, then knowledge of the pharmacology of hallucinogens consists of trying to understand the mechanisms by which this knowledge itself is produced. It could be said that the pharmacology of hallucinogens is actually a philosophical discipline that is studied through scientific methods commonly used in psychology and biology.

Pharmacology is the science that studies the effects of drugs on the body. In the case of hallucinogenic drugs, there are two subdisciplines of particular interest: psychopharmacology, which is the study of effects on behavior, and neuropharmacology, which is the study of effects on the nervous system. In the first, the study is carried out using tools developed by psychology such as psychometric questionnaires, and in the latter, with tools from neurology (the study of receptors and mechanisms of action). It is a complex science, since relating psychological processes with neurobiological mechanisms is not an easy task. All this aside from the risk of trying to explain phenomena belonging to different levels of analysis, one with the other's categories. The most current example is that of the famous default mode network construct, so popular in current neuroscience in general, and in that of hallucinogens in particular. I leave it to the reader to get to the corresponding part in this book, to see how easy it is to fall into this type of bias, and how the author solves it so accurately. And similarly, many other examples that only a person with mixed training in psychology and pharmacology, together with great experience in the empirical field, can draw our attention to and clarify.

In this sense, Genís has been able to place each explanation at its corresponding level of analysis, thus avoiding the reductionisms that are so typical of this field. In a context in which biomedicine is dominating research agendas and budgets, even though its clinical application is extremely limited compared to other approaches, based mainly on public health or social and community practices, the author wanted to reflect on its scope and limitations and devote some final chapters to the reduction of risks in the use of hallucinogens and the recognition that should be given to traditional societies, which are ultimately the discoverers of many of these compounds. If in our society we establish mind-brain relationships in accordance with the parallel advances of both neurobiology and psychology, a field of extremely interesting value will be one to connect these disciplines with traditional Indigenous knowledge in relation to hallucinogenic plants and compounds. In his essential book *Consilience: The Unity of Knowledge* (1998), the recently deceased biologist Edward O. Wilson already pointed in that direction, precisely using ayahuasca and one of its best-known cultural expressions, the art of the Peruvian mestizo painter Pablo Amaringo, as an example.

In short, what we have here is an a priori arduous field, which becomes attractive when we understand that its concepts reveal the keys that will allow us to go deeper and deeper into the knowledge of what is the essence of the human being. Hallucinogens, as writers like Aldous Huxley or chemists like Alexander Shulgin have said, are incomparable tools for learning about mind-brain relationships. And the discipline that deals with this study is pharmacology. The last twenty years have been vertiginous in terms of the development and progress in knowledge of the pharmacology of hallucinogens, but this knowledge is only present in scientific journals; it has not reached the general public. That is why this book is so pertinent at this time. We needed a translator, a compiler who could bring what is in that inaccessible world of scientific literature down to Earth, a feat that can only be achieved satisfactorily if the one doing it can masterfully combine scientific knowledge and humanistic sensibility in such a way that scientific abstraction can be understood in its social context. In the case of Genís Ona, these two types of knowledge coexist, allowing him to move away from literal and reductionist explanations, without avoiding the complexity of the phenomena and making precise interpretations of the data.

Writing a book like this was no easy task, if one did not want to betray the goal of making it for all audiences. My congratulations to the author. I think he can feel satisfied with the result. If an intellectually restless person seeks to know the processes that mediate between matter and spirit, how these processes have been discovered, what philosophical and therapeutic implications they have, and, above all, to update on the level of knowledge that is now available about them and their relationship to hallucinogenic or psychedelic drugs, this is your book. I can be nothing but proud for having been asked to write a foreword by the author, the only independent researcher in Spain who is currently administering hallucinogens in clinical settings to study their pharmacology and therapeutic potential. And someone who, in addition to being a tireless collaborator, is a good friend. Genís's resumé, by the way, in terms of scientific publications in impactful journals, exceeds the average researcher, and more so in a field as complicated as psychedelic research has been, until relatively recently. This book is therefore another small success in his already brilliant career, of which

I am sure we will all feel proud in the future, even more than we feel now. Researchers like him are role models for this coming generation, of which he is a part, to lead the way in psychedelic research.

JOSÉ CARLOS BOUSO, PH.D.,
SCIENTIFIC DIRECTOR OF ICEERS

JOSÉ CARLOS BOUSO is a clinical psychologist with a Ph.D. in pharmacology. He developed his scientific activities while at the Universidad Autónoma de Madrid, the Instituto de Investigación Biomédica IIB-Sant Pau de Barcelona, and the Instituto Hospital del Mar de Investigaciones Médicas de Barcelona (IMIM). During this time, he developed studies about the therapeutic effects of MDMA (ecstasy) and psychopharmacological studies on the acute and neuropsychiatric long-term effects of many substances, both synthetic and of plant origin. As the Scientific Director at ICEERS, the International Center for Ethnobotanical Education, Research, and Service, José Carlos coordinates studies on the potential benefits of psychoactive plants, principally cannabis, ayahuasca, and ibogaine, with the goal of improving public health. He is coauthor of numerous scientific papers and several book chapters. He is also a member of the Medical Anthropology Research Center (MARC) at the Universitat Rovira i Virgili in Tarragona, visiting professor in the mental health program at the Faculty of Medicine of the University of São Paulo in Riberão Preto, Brazil, and vice-president of the Society of Clinical Endocannabinology (SEC).

Preface

The first time I came in contact with psychedelic drugs, I knew instantly that my life had changed. I knew I was embarking on a journey of no return, on a ship sailing toward unknown territories, and I would never find a port in which to rest, since few mysteries resist the advancement of knowledge as much as the characteristic alterations of consciousness induced by these substances. However, despite this certainty, I suppose that one sometimes feels the call and follows it, without looking back. And it is paradoxical, to say the least, that some substances called *psychedelics* (a word formed by *psykhe*, soul, breath, and *dēlos*, show, reveal) contain mysteries that are so complicated to unravel. Nevertheless, although this contradiction seems evident here, the truth is that a large part of what concerns the human organism and the action external molecules can exert on it still lives in buried treasures that await, unhurriedly, to be discovered.

Personally, I began to study psychedelic drugs from a psychological point of view, obviously thinking that the most important thing about them would be their psychological effects. However, it did not take long for me to realize that, in order to approach them, it was necessary to widen the scope a little more. I then became interested in what anthropologists and ethnologists had to say about them, through descriptions of exotic journeys and literally mind-blowing adventures. Learning this perspective seemed one of the fundamental pillars for anyone who approaches these drugs, since it is of course necessary to place them in their historical context and understand the ways in which different cultures have used them, especially with regard to their communal and spiritual use. Later on, I drifted into a much more biomedical arena, for various reasons, although I would highlight the fact that I perceived the need to study these drugs from as serious and respectable a perspective as possible. I was also aware that there was much more to be done in medical-scientific settings that, despite their robustness and seriousness, were actually the least understood in the field. I therefore studied neurotoxicology and neuropsychopharmacology applied to animal research, and later pursued studies in human pharmacology, subsequently undertaking a doctorate in health, psychology, and psychiatry. Thus, at the time of this writing, I believe I have some experience and expertise in the fields of psychology, anthropology, and pharmacology that allow me to better understand what psychedelic drugs do to our minds. However, I still don't understand everything.

Despite not understanding everything, I dared to write this book, perhaps so that others could also reach the same conclusion. In fact, I wish we could all get there! One comes across many books on neuroscience, psychopharmacology, and popular science in general, launching bold statements without foundation or proclaiming supposed absolute certainties on issues that are still not very well understood. Nevertheless, we must not forget that science is a method of obtaining knowledge that works with provisional knowledge, where hypotheses or theories are generated that often have little to do with reality. We often settle for these simplistic or reductionist explanations of complex phenomena, and there is a reason for this: we want certainties. Our brains are prepared to build schemes, models of our environment, with the intention of predicting, as much as possible, future situations in which our lives may be in danger. But sometimes this gets out of hand. We cannot understand everything. Let the person holding this book know that they will not find certainties here. In this book we will navigate together through uncertainty, which should be the true defining characteristic of the scientific enterprise. It is only when we position ourselves in the awareness of not knowing that we begin to learn. I daresay we should cultivate this state more often.

Certainly, when we talk about the pharmacology of psychedelic drugs, we find ourselves in a highly complex field. This discipline should answer questions such as: Why does this molecule cause this primate to think of itself as God? To answer, you must first ask yourself: How does the human brain convert chemicals into thoughts? The answer to this question is still as far away as the horizon itself. However, despite these limitations, the pharmacological knowledge of these drugs has advanced extraordinarily in recent decades, and although we cannot answer essential questions, we can answer other tangential ones, which is not trivial.

The rise of psychedelic drugs, not only as possible therapeutic tools, but also as valuable tools to better understand functions as complex as consciousness itself, is already unstoppable. Researchers from all over the world are immersed in this search like never before, and the many possibilities are hardly imaginable. What was unthinkable just fifteen or twenty years ago is not only happening today but is exceeding all expectations. Ambitious research programs are being financed by governments and billionaire investments in the development of medicines based on psychedelic drugs, with the approval of the most important regulatory agencies. It would not be surprising if shortly after this book is published, the use of psilocybin or 3,4-methylenedioxymethamphetamine (MDMA) for the treatment of certain psychological disorders is approved, or that some decisive step is taken in basic research in neuroscience thanks to a psychedelic compound. Not even the most powerful psychedelic drug imaginable could show us the exciting future that awaits.

It is foreseeable that this new wave of studies and research with psychedelics will also lead to advances in the knowledge of adjacent fields. From ICEERS (International Center for Ethnobotanical Education, Research, and Service), one of the organizations in which I work, we organized the third international conference on ayahuasca in 2019, and to my surprise, during most of the conference, everything but ayahuasca seemed to be discussed! There were sessions on the sustainability of ecosystems like the Amazon, art, biodiversity, Indigenous communities, history, human rights, and colonialism. For me, the intellectual interest in psychedelic drugs has also aroused a voracious interest in the pharmacology of natural products and in the general functioning of the nervous system and our minds. This is why I encourage my readers to enter this field of study with enthusiasm and an open mind, because it is very likely that you will end up getting hooked on other fields that have nothing to do, at first glance, with psychedelic drugs. The transdisciplinary nature of this field that defines psychedelics is perhaps its best attribute, and the new information that we receive almost daily about psychedelics is a gift we must take advantage of and exploit to its fullest.

I remember when I was in high school, I must have been about twelve or thirteen years old, I had not tried any drugs, except for a little glass of wine with my family and a puff here and there of a cigarette that someone had procured somehow. However, I had already read Antonio Escohotado, Thomas Szasz, Albert Hofmann, Stanislav Grof, Aldous Huxley, and Jack Kerouac! So the subject of "drugs" was beginning to look like a pretty fascinating world to me. Back then, in my high school natural sciences textbook, I found a couple of pages that covered "drugs." As soon as I started reading the content I started to freak out. It was nothing but alarmist information or directly implausible fallacies. I was stunned. Much more than that: I was deeply incensed at the thought that my generation, and many others before and perhaps after, would be confronted with this pack of lies and thus exposed to information that simply wasn't true. How was that possible? It took less than a few hours, I think, for me to get to work. I made a list of all the statements that were wrong, false, or at least required some nuance, adding the correct information to each and the sources from which I had obtained the information. I attached the list to a letter addressed to the publishers at Santillana, in which I strongly suggested that they correct the content in future editions of the book on natural sciences, and I sent it by post to their headquarters. A couple of weeks later I was summoned to the office of the headmaster. There, with him, were two lawyers from Santillana. They let me know that they had not liked the aforementioned letter very much and that they could even report me to the authorities (truth be told, I do not remember why, but I may have asked them to modify the content of the books a little *too* emphatically). In short, they forced me to write another letter in which I retracted what I had said in the previous one. Right then and there, handwritten. And the matter was settled. I was a scared kid who didn't know anything about life, I didn't do things right, and at the time I had no other choice. But I'm not that kid anymore.

This book is, in part, a crystallization of that premature desire to combat disinformation. I hope that it can help many people receive the upcoming future of psychedelic drugs in a way that is informed, safe, free from prejudice, and, of course, open to what we do not yet know. I have decided to include two appendices at the end of the book, which I highly recommend readers peruse. In particular, I suggest taking a look at the glossary of technical or specific terms to facilitate a smooth reading experience without the need to pause and search for the meanings of certain terms. There are also "References for Further Study" sections at the end of some chapters so that readers can delve further into the subject matter.

I would like to thank all the people who have made this book possible: first of all, the fantastic team at Inner Traditions, for its enthusiasm and for this unique opportunity. Thank you so much, especially to Elizabeth, for your care and patience throughout the process. It has been a pleasure to be accompanied by your team and collaborators.

I am grateful to all the teachers who have accompanied me in my academic learning. To Pepita, Salvador Escudé, Manel, Rocaspana, Pere Joan, Inés, Teresa, Santafé, Jordi—thanks for everything.

I'd also like to thank my mother and father, for loving me to the best of their ability and always being there for me.

Thank you, Aryan Sarparast, for your invaluable assistance, your trust, and the compassion you embody!

Thanks to the fantastic team at ICEERS, my second family, who has always believed in me and offered me so many opportunities and unforgettable moments.

Thank you, Bou, for being my mentor and friend and for all that you've helped me learn.

Thank you, Eva, for joining me in the process of writing this book, for your careful reading of the proofs, and for your wise suggestions and corrections—but above all, thank you for accompanying me in this life and for your love. *T'estimo, mor.*

My regards and gratitude also to those who are no longer here, for teaching me what is really important.

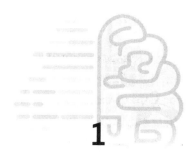

1

Brief Introduction to Pharmacology

The most important result of a rational inquiry into nature is, therefore, to establish the unity and harmony of this stupendous mass of force and matter.

ALEXANDER VON HUMBOLDT

Pharmacology is a word associated with a certain field of study that is quite technical. Pharmacology tends to be understood as a complicated science, dedicated to the study of medicines and their effects, a subject that is certainly not part of our daily lives. We do not argue with our friends or relatives about pharmacokinetics[1] or about the binding of this or that substance to receptors. However, drugs, in their most general sense, are widely present in our society. And not only in ours, as we find evidence of the use of drugs in all human societies from their written history. Isn't it strange, then, that the knowledge regarding these widely used products is not accessible to everyone? This book aims to do just that. I will not try to make the reader confirm the general opinion that pharmacology is something complicated. On the

---

1. The study of pharmacology is concerned with the absorption, distribution, metabolism, and elimination of a drug in the body. It can be said that pharmacokinetics studies what happens to a drug from the time it enters an organism until it is totally eliminated. It is summarized in the phrase "What does the body do to the drug?"

contrary: I hope to make the reader familiar with it in a much more friendly way.

The term *psychedelic* is used to refer to a group of substances and products[2] that produce effects that are, precisely, psychedelic. These can be synthetic (LSD, MDMA) or natural (mushrooms of the *Psilocybe* or *Amanita* genus, ayahuasca), and the truth is that it is difficult to define these psychedelic effects. It is generally characterized by distortions in the senses (you may hear better, in more detail, or a wall may be perceived to move as if it were "breathing"), changes in thought (may increase speed of thought or creativity), or very sudden and intense changes in mood (burst into inconsolable tears one minute and be in a fit of laughter the next). Peak experiences, using Abraham Maslow's terminology, are also frequent at high doses. These are experiences that allow us to transcend the usual perception of oneself as a person and our environment. Maslow (1908–1970) was an American psychologist who founded humanistic psychology, and when he spoke of peak experiences he emphasized harmony. In these states it is usual to feel in harmony with oneself and with existence. The perception of time and space dims and a deep sense of well-being is heightened.

In short, the aim of this book on psychedelic pharmacology is to explain how psychedelic substances work, how they can have such dramatic effects on perception and thought, and what these substances do to our brain. These are some of the questions that we will try to answer from the perspective of pharmacology.

ETYMOLOGICAL ORIGINS

In this book we do not think it is necessary to delve much into the etymological origin of the word *psychedelic*, since other books address

---

2. At this point, we must differentiate the terms *substance* and *product*. In English, the term *substance* is used to refer to synthetic or semisynthetic active principles (LSD, psilocybin), while *product* refers to the natural source from which they may or may not be extracted. In this way, we can say that ayahuasca is a product from which substances (DMT) can be extracted, or that MDMA or ecstasy is a very powerful substance.

it in greater detail. However, it is worth mentioning its literal meaning, as it is certainly interesting. It is formed from the Greek words *psykhe* (soul, mind) and *dēlos* (manifest, reveal). Therefore, everything we call psychedelic would be that which helps a person reveal one's own soul or one's own mind.

As for the origin of the word *pharmacology*, we are going to stop a little longer to comment on its fascinating etymology. First of all, in classical Greek *phármakon* means "drug." Far from the clear pejorative connotations that this word currently has in our culture, originally the term was much more neutral, and therefore more complex. In fact, an almost identical and probably earlier term is *pharmakós*, which means "sacrificial lamb." Pharmakós was the name given to a person who was going to undergo some kind of sacrifice. It must be remembered that these sacrifices were not always lethal; it could be exile, stoning, or other tormenting punishments; although the term referred to all the "victims" of these practices, all of them constituted part of a kind of purification ritual. When the community was hit by catastrophes or droughts, or individuals fell gravely ill, these events were interpreted as deregulations in the delicate balance between humans and gods, which evidenced the need to readjust said harmony by offering the gods the *pharmakoi* (plural of pharmakós), who carried all the impurities (or miasma) of the people. In other words, they would gather and concentrate "all that was bad" to later destroy it. But what relationship did the pharmakoi have with drugs or phármakon? Although it is mere conjecture, some authors suggest that, once sacrifices and other practices gave way to classical Greek rationality—including Hippocratic medicine—by the fifth century BCE, the personification of the ills of the community for subsequent sacrifice was no longer considered essential. In fact, this magical act came to be conceived as a practice typical of charlatans. The pharmakós, the poor victim who would be sacrificed, became an impersonal phármakon (a botanical preparation, for example) capable of "purifying" a body without the need for another being to succumb in the process.

Interestingly, another similar word in Greek (although its relationship to *phármakon* is less clear) is *pharmasso*, which means "to temper iron," that is, when red hot iron is submerged in cold water. "To temper" has an unequivocal meaning in psychological terms, being synonymous with soothing, calming. In this sense, it may be that at some point the effects of the phármakon (at least when substances such as opium were used) were associated with the action of "tempering" the iron. Likewise, another close concept is *pharmak*, which is formed by the first part (*phar*) that could derive from the Indo-European root *bher* (which means "to move," "to carry") and the second part (*mak*), also from an Indo-European root, which means "power." In that a case, the possibly oldest root of the term *drug* (phármakon) would be referring to a substance with the "power" of "moving" (impurities).

Regarding the term *phármakon* itself, its meaning was not limited exclusively to the concept of drug, as we have seen. Phármakon could refer to medicines, poisons, or remedies. This is because sometimes the difference between a remedy and a poison, so (supposedly) evident today, was not so clear. As Paracelsus[3] would say centuries later, the difference may lie in the dosage. Therefore, the word *phármakon* did not have the same negative connotations that the word *drug* currently has for us. It referred only to a chemical vehicle used to intervene in the functions of an organism.

MAIN PHARMACOLOGICAL CONCEPTS

To talk about the pharmacological properties of psychedelic substances or products, I need to mention a few somewhat technical concepts. We will find them throughout the book, so I dedicate the following lines to briefly describe them. Nevertheless, at the end of this book you can find a glossary of words and technical concepts that you can consult at any time.

---

3. Born in 1493, Paracelsus was a Swiss alchemist, doctor, astrologer, and expert in toxicology. Paracelsus was in fact the name that he himself invented, and it means "equal or similar to Celsus," who was one of the most influential Roman physicians who lived in the first century CE.

Nervous System

Before we get started with pharmacology itself, it is necessary to briefly introduce the "playing field," that is to say, the place where all the reactions or processes that I am going to mention will take place. It is our nervous system. It is made up of the central nervous system (CNS) and the autonomic nervous system (ANS).

The CNS is made up of the brain and the spinal cord. Both structures are protected by the skull and the spinal column, respectively, which already informs us of their crucial importance. The CNS is where most of the body's functions will be coordinated, and where we find the structures without which few of these functions would be possible. Forming part of the brain we find the cerebrum, cerebellum, and medulla oblongata. The brain is where functions as complex as the integration of sensory information, information processing, or emotional processing, among many others, are carried out. It is made up of two zones clearly distinguishable by their colors: gray matter and white matter. The first corresponds to sets of neuronal cell bodies, while white matter corresponds to nerve fibers that connect these neuronal bodies. Higher functions, such as reasoning or planning, seem to be located mostly in the cerebral cortex, a broad mantle about 3 mm thick that covers the entire surface of the brain. Regions or neurons that lie under this cortex are called subcortical.

The evolutionarily older regions of the brain are those that lie deeper and are called limbic structures or limbic brain, while the regions that are more recent, from an evolutionary point of view, are closer to the cortex, being the neocortex, the most recently developed structure. It should be noted that, apart from these regions and structures, the brain is an organ endowed with remarkable plasticity, so that it "constructs" itself in correspondence with the development of the individual and their experiences.

The cerebellum has typically been associated with motor functions, although it also performs notable cognitive and sensory functions. The medulla oblongata is located at the base of the brain and is a connecting area between the brain and the spinal cord. Also found in this structure

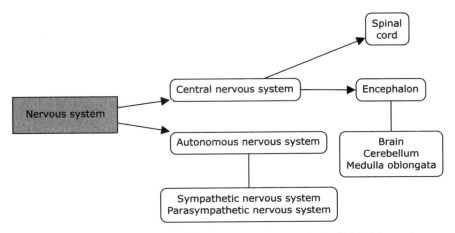

Figure 1. Schematic view of the nervous system. It is divided into the central nervous system (CNS) and the autonomic nervous system (ANS). The CNS includes the spinal cord and the brain, the latter including the cerebrum, cerebellum, and medulla oblongata. The ANS includes the sympathetic and parasympathetic nervous systems.

are many nuclei responsible for automatic body functions, such as breathing or heart rate. In the medulla oblongata, there is an important opiate receptor density, and that is why an overdose of opiates can risk the life of the user, because, if the activity of these nuclei is inhibited with sufficient intensity, automatic processes like the ones mentioned above can be interrupted.

The ANS is called autonomous precisely because it coordinates functions that are generally beyond the reach of our will or even our consciousness. It is basically made up of the nerves that connect the CNS with the rest of our organism, so it can send and receive signals from any point in our body. It is made up of the sympathetic and parasympathetic nervous systems.

The sympathetic nervous system is mainly related to the sudden activation of our body in situations of need. When we are faced with some dangerous or threatening situation, it is this part of our nervous system that activates the necessary resources to succeed. It is responsible, for example, for emptying the bladder, for sending more blood to the extremities so

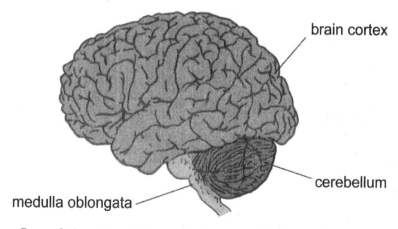

brain cortex

cerebellum

medulla oblongata

Figure 2. Location of the cerebral cortex (which actually covers the entire surface of the brain), the cerebellum, at the back, and the medulla oblongata, which is at the base of the brain.

you can run farther, and for releasing more adrenaline to better withstand possible pain. In short, it prepares the body for fight-or-flight reactions.

The parasympathetic nervous system has the opposite function. Its activation is associated with increased relaxation or the induction of a resting state, for example, by slowing the heart rate.

Neurons, Synapses, and Action Potentials

Neurons are the specific cells of the nervous system. Although they are one of the most complex known entities in the universe, fortunately neurons, and the small pieces of which they are made, can be understood relatively simply. For starters, the neuron can be either on or off, like a switch. Those are its only two states; there is no middle ground.

The function of the neuron is to receive and send information. Its structure is precisely and elegantly designed to fulfill this purpose. It contains three fundamental parts: the cell body, the dendrites, and the axon. The cell body is quite similar to any other cell, and shares some of its structures, such as the cell nucleus. Dendrites are small appendages that extend from the cell body and undertake the mission of receiving information from their direct environment. As for the axons, these are

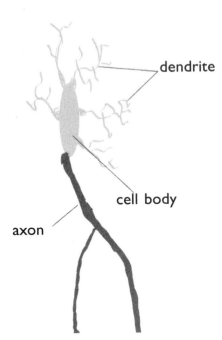

dendrite

cell body

axon

Figure 3. Basic diagram of a neuron.

much longer appendages, specifically dealing with the transmission of information to other neurons or cells. Sometimes these axons can be long enough to span the distance between the spinal cord and the toes. The blue whale, for example, needs a 9-m axon to be able to move its baleen.

Neurons are organized in local circuits or networks that are also in constant communication with distant regions, so that it is quite similar to our current road networks: multiple local or regional road circuits that are also widely connected by highways and motorways with distant locations.

When a cell body receives information from another cell (usually, but not exclusively, from its dendrites), a synapse is produced. A synapse is nothing more than the intercellular connection that allows for effective communication. It is estimated that each neuron is somewhat directly connected to one thousand other neurons, although this is a difficult number to estimate. It should be added that the mechanism by which this communication occurs is known as action potentials. Continuing with the highway metaphor, the synapse would be the asphalt, while the action potential is the vehicle that travels on it. Let's explain action potentials in further detail.

An action potential is the "shot" of electrical energy that allows neuronal communication.

All neurons are covered by a membrane that not only separates the inside of the neuron from the outside but is also electrically charged. Most of the time the inside of the neuron has a slightly more negative charge than the outside (−70 mV). This slight negativity defines the resting state of the neuron (remember the switch). When it is off, there are also higher concentrations of potassium in relation to those of sodium and calcium, inside with respect to the outside.

When the neuron is not at rest and turns "on," a change occurs in some of its properties that allows small amounts of sodium (which has a positive charge) to access its interior. The result is that the inside of the neuron is progressively more positive than the outside (up to about +40 mV). It is at this moment that the neuron enters the so-called depolarization phase (precisely because there is a change in polarity) and an action potential is produced. Within a tenth of a second, the action potential fades, repolarization occurs, and the neuron returns to a negative, resting state. Looking at figure 4 as you read these lines can help you better understand the entire process.

This action potential should be explained in the context of a network of neurons that are interconnected, because when an action potential occurs it is not located in a particular neuron, but rather extends between all neurons that have a direct connection. After all, we need to understand this process as the transmission of an electrical impulse and, as such, it will travel[4] in every possible direction and for as long as

---

4. Namely, nerve impulses produced by action potentials can travel at speeds of over 100 meters per second.

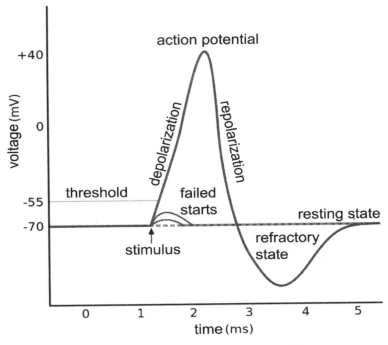

Figure 4. Phases of the action potential.

it finds a way to do so. When the nerve impulse generated by the action potential reaches other neurons, it will cause the release of neurotransmitters, giving rise to subsequent cascades of effects.

Pharmacokinetics and Pharmacodynamics

These are two concepts widely used in the field of pharmacology. Although they may seem like complicated concepts, their meaning is actually quite simple. Pharmacokinetics is dedicated to studying what the body does to the drug, while pharmacodynamics studies what the drug does to the body. The order in which these two concepts are presented is important, as it follows a logical sequence that helps to understand their meaning. Pharmacokinetics, which is what happens to the drug when it enters our body, is always mentioned first, and pharmacodynamics, which consists of the study of all the effects the drug has on the body, second. Simply put, only once it has been absorbed and metabolized do we notice its effects (relaxing, analgesic, or psychedelic, depending on the type of drug or substance). Pharmacodynamics is therefore something that necessarily follows pharmacokinetics.

Pharmacokinetics is generally classified into different areas of study that make up the acronym RADME (release, absorption, distribution, metabolism, and excretion), which we will also see later in this book. As we can see, these phases describe the entire course of action of a drug from the time we ingest it to the time we excrete it. We study how a drug is released (a factor that will vary depending on whether the drug is administered orally or injected, for example), how it is absorbed (absorption may vary even among pills that are ingested orally, since this depends on many factors, including the acidic or basic characteristics of the drug, also known as its pH), how it is distributed in the body (that is, what diffusion capabilities it demonstrates and which tissues or organs it is able to reach), how it is metabolized (via the liver, kidney, or other mechanisms), and how it is eliminated or excreted (mainly in the urine, although it can also be excreted through the skin, lungs, breast milk, and other avenues).

All these phases are studied by means of complicated parameters and equations, which, of course, we will not get into. Still, an important parameter that needs to be introduced, and one that we will see often in this book, is the half-life, generally represented as "T1/2." The half-life of a drug is calculated in hours or minutes and represents the time required for the concentration of a given drug in the plasma to be reduced by half. In other words, if a drug has a half-life of two hours, such as ibuprofen, and it has a concentration of 400 mg[5] in blood plasma at a given time, after two hours the concentration will be reduced to 200 mg, in two more hours to 100 mg, and so on. The faster a drug is "cleared," primarily through the liver or kidneys, the shorter the half-life of a drug, so drugs that take longer to metabolize and eliminate

---

5. This number is not random. Ibuprofen doses are usually administered in 600-mg tablets, but they are not fully absorbed. A considerable fraction, between 25 percent and 50 percent, will not pass into the blood plasma, so that a reasonable plasma concentration after an hour of having taken 600 mg of ibuprofen would be about 400 mg.

will have longer half-lives. Generally, lipophilic drugs, known as such because of their great affinity to fats, are those with the longest half-life times, as they bind to fats, releasing fractions of the drug much more slowly and continuously. In theory, the body is considered to be free of a drug when ten half-lives of the drug have passed, whatever that may be, since at that point only 1/1,000 of the original dose will remain in circulation. In figure 5, we can see how the plasma concentration of a drug rises after acute intake and is progressively eliminated.

Pharmacodynamics is made up of all the effects drugs have on the body. All biological or physiological modifications are studied in this area of pharmacology. This includes desired modifications (primary effects), such as the analgesic effect of paracetamol (Tylenol), as well as unwanted modifications, which are known as secondary or toxic effects. The study of the pharmacodynamics of drugs soon emphasizes the importance of dosage. In general, at higher doses, the effects of a drug will be more powerful or notable, until reaching a "ceiling" that can no longer be overcome, regardless of how much the dosage is increased. Furthermore, as the dose increases, although the desired effects may not increase, undesired effects do tend to increase.

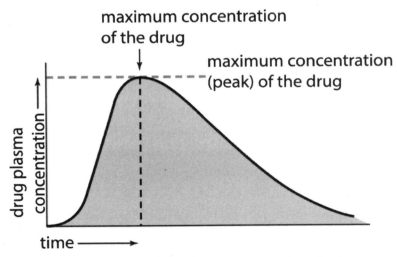

Figure 5. Variation of the plasma concentration of a drug.
After ingestion, its concentration rises rapidly, falling progressively
after reaching the maximum plasma concentration.

Regarding the study of psychedelic drugs, the methods of pharmacodynamics are, in most cases, the same as those used in other drugs. These include electroencephalograms or neuroimaging techniques while the person is under the influence of a substance, measuring their blood pressure, heart rate, running blood tests, or using other parameters. However, due to the intense and particular effects that these substances have on the mind, researchers in this field have devised a series of methods to also evaluate the psychological aspects of these effects. In clinical trial contexts, this has been carried out mainly in two different ways: through validated psychometric questionnaires (a typical questionnaire made up of a series of items in which typical experiences associated with psychedelic effects are described, and the person is asked to answer the degree to which they have experienced these phenomena while under these effects), and through Visual Analog Scales or VAS. These scales are frequently used to measure pain, for example, when someone asks you the typical question: "On a scale from 1 to 10, how much does it hurt?" In this case, the researchers designed a list of typical psychedelic experiences, with a horizontal line of 10 cm below each experience, along which the subject is asked to draw a small vertical line depending on the intensity of their experience with each phenomenon. A vertical line that is closer to the beginning of the horizontal line means

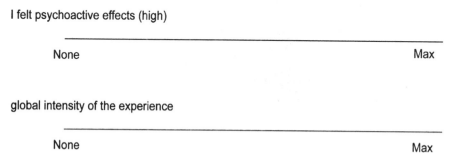

I felt psychoactive effects (high)

None   Max

global intensity of the experience

None   Max

Figure 6. Examples of VAS, or Visual Analog Scales. In the horizontal lines, the subject has to make a small vertical line at some point on the line according to their own experience. For example, in the first case, if the subject experiences very intense psychoactive effects then the vertical line will be drawn toward the end.

the intensity was low, while one toward the end of the horizontal line means the intensity was higher; see figure 6.

The most curious example, to say the least, of an evaluation of pharmacodynamics that I can recall occurred at the Hospital de la Santa Creu i Sant Pau, in Barcelona. I was working on my master's thesis with Dr. Jordi Riba, who had put me in charge of the recruitment and daily management of a clinical trial with salvinorin-A, the active ingredient of the plant *Salvia divinorum* and one of the most powerful psychedelics out there. The study tried to find the "ideal dose" for use in humans, so volunteers were to be exposed to different doses of pure salvinorin-A (0, 250, 500, 750, and 1,000 micrograms). The doses were given in that order, but the subjects were told that they would be given at random, so we could also observe possible suggestive effects within the context (although there was virtually no one who reported experiencing effects when given 0 mg). Salvinorin-A was administered by inhalation, using a blowtorch to burn the contents of a flask covered with foil so that no one could see the contents. Each subject was "trained" to perform an uninterrupted inhalation for thirty seconds, which would guarantee that all the vapor from the combustion would be absorbed. The experimental sessions started by having the person stretch out on a bed, then we would perform the breathing training and bring over the flask, at which point Jordi would light the blowtorch, the person would inhale all its contents, stretch out again, and begin their particular psychedelic journey while I watched the entire scene and assisted Jordi with anything he needed (providing him with materials, removing the table where the flask was sitting, holding the legs of a participant in the middle of a delirium while Jordi held their arms and torso, and the like). Salvinorin-A induces powerful psychoactive effects in less than a minute, and they also end very quickly, usually within ten to fifteen minutes, so it's a very intense but very brief experience. Jordi had a Visual Analog Scale of a single question he asked the subjects out loud thirty seconds after the end of inhalation, that is, one minute after inhalation began. The question was simply: "Rate the intensity of the experience from 0 to 100," to which the subjects had to answer with a number, also out loud. Well, it turns out that when we administered the highest dose (1,000 mg) none of the subjects responded. They didn't hear Jordi. They simply were no longer there! When that happened, Jordi would write down "100" and look at me smiling.

Neurotransmitters

There is a wide variety of substances in our body called neurotransmitters. Their function is basically to transmit information from one cell to another, which is why they are also often called "messengers." They regulate physiological functions such as heartbeat, movements, sleep, and modulating a person's mood and how they react to different stimuli in their environment.

Among the most well-known neurotransmitters are serotonin (abbreviated as 5-HT) and dopamine. We can classify neurotransmitters according to the basic function they perform when they are released. In this way, we find excitatory neurotransmitters, such as acetylcholine or epinephrine, and inhibitors, such as GABA or serotonin. In a big mixed bag we can place the so-called modulatory neurotransmitters, which play different roles in the body's functions. For example, endorphins, which are endogenous opioids, deal with reducing pain signals in the event of injuries, blows, stressful situations, and the like.

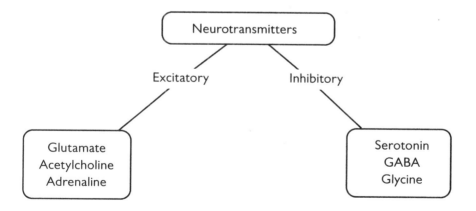

Figure 7. Basic classification and examples of neurotransmitters. Mainly, we can find excitatory (glutamate, acetylcholine, and adrenaline) and inhibitory (serotonin, GABA, and glycine) neurotransmitters.

Excitatory neurotransmitters will have an effect mainly of activation or hyperactivation of the tissues that contain the receptors to which they are going to be bound. This occurs mainly by increasing the frequency of action potentials. Similarly, inhibitory neurotransmitters reduce the frequency with which these action potentials occur.

Receptors

One of the topics that we will see most frequently in this book is the one related to the action of psychedelic drugs on certain receptors. But what are receptors? We can define receptors as proteins or groups of proteins found on the cell membrane. Cells are like small rooms full of structures and chemical substances, which are also in constant communication with other cells, whether they are near or far. If your understanding of cells was that these were isolated entities working autonomously, forget that image. The functioning of the cells is more like a great, gigantic swarm working in unison and constantly communicating. To satisfy this "social" nature, cells have a complex communication system, in which receptors are essential.

Receptors are so named precisely because they "receive" information from the environment. The most common way of receiving information is through molecules that bind to these receptors. Thus, as if it were a messenger, when a certain molecule binds to the receptor of a cell, the activity or function of this cell is modified based on the information received. We will see how this happens later.

Whether or not molecules can bind to receptors will depend on their degree of affinity for said receptors. In two words, and simplifying a lot, if the structure of the molecule "fits well" with the protein structure of the receptor, then it will bind more easily. If the structures are very different, said molecule will not be able to interact with the receptor and will simply not adhere to it. We have to understand that if psychedelic drugs such as LSD or ayahuasca produce psychedelic effects, it is thanks to the fact that the molecules they contain can bind to certain receptors in our body. This fact may be surprising, given that, generally and broadly speaking, the receptors that we have in our bodies respond

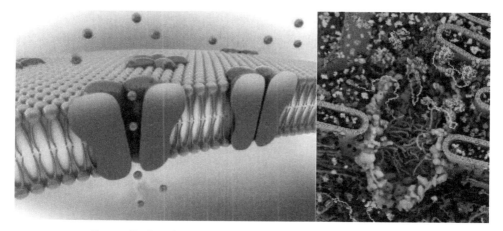

Figure 8. Graphic representation of brain receptors (*left*)
and a real image of a receptor (*right*). (See also color plate 1.)

to their own molecules. So why do psychedelics as potent as salvinorin-A or LSD (which is man-made) bind to our receptors?

The answer to this question is simpler than you might think. And no, it's not that evolution wants us to get high. To understand it, we have to step back and see the scenario from a historical point of view. First of all, it must be said that millions of years ago, when the plant kingdom was born with the first mosses and then began to diversify into increasingly complex and resistant plants, the resources that these plants had at their disposal were extremely limited. Of course they had sunlight, but the inorganic materials that they could access through their roots were scarce. As a consequence, in order to save as much energy as possible, plants began to design a large number of strategies to synthesize the chemicals they needed, by using the small traces of molecules that they had inside or closest to them in the environment. Thus, a large number of chemical components that shared very similar nuclei and structures began to fill the chemical arsenal of the plant kingdom.

Some of these chemicals were not designed to meet the essential needs of plants but to attack other living things that wanted to eat them. These compounds are called secondary metabolites, precisely because they are not essential for plant survival but are synthesized exclusively for attacking other organisms and for other communication functions. If we remember the hostile environment in which these plants lived (and still live), you will think that a poor little fern only needed an herbivore 20 times its size to come and eat it. Well, plants could get out of such situations thanks to these chemicals. The catch was getting it right the first time. If the chemical did not effectively bind to the animal's receptors, dramatically modifying its behavior or its vital functions, it would mean missing the mark and, therefore, being eaten. So in addition to having a fairly diverse arsenal of secondary metabolites, these compounds were also specially designed to bind to a large number of different receptors. They weren't selective darts. They were fragmentation grenades.

Some of these chemicals are coagulants, some are paralyzing, and some get you high. Intoxication is as old as life itself. After all, we are dealing with an alteration of the normal functioning of the nervous system: just what those plants tried to achieve to defend themselves. A romantic and highly unlikely idea would be that, in the case of plants that synthesized psychoactive compounds, the way to defend themselves was to induce in their predator a super powerful mystical experience that would remind them of the interconnectedness of all forms of life and the infinite love that had created them, as can happen with high doses of some psychedelics. However, as we've said, this is more than unlikely. In the first place, if that predator is starving, what the plant in question needs is to drive it away, producing much more aversive stimuli than something that merely generates the thought "Wow, everything is so beautiful." Secondly, with the knowledge we currently have, it is impossible to conceive of any member of the plant kingdom having ever had the ability to understand the inner life of beings belonging to other kingdoms. And, thirdly, the insects and small herbivores for which these chemicals were designed (no, they were not designed for hominids) probably did not have the complex psychological experiences that humans have when ingesting them. Surely they had totally different effects. A good example is the cannabinoids produced by the *Cannabis sativa* plant. Insects do not have cannabinoid receptors; therefore, these substances do not usually have a direct effect on them. However, cannabinoids inhibit defense mechanisms of insects against other secondary metabolites, and therefore they do not have the function of inducing a high, but rather of increasing the toxic capability of other compounds present in the plant.

Some especially attentive and thoughtful reader may wonder: "But why do we still have receptors capable of interacting with these compounds if, at the time they were synthesized, nothing remotely resembling a monkey existed on Earth?" And it would be a legitimate question. The separation of millions and millions of years of evolution between the synthesis of these compounds and the appearance of human beings would be a sufficient lapse of time to think that, at some point, the progressively more complex forms of animal life would simply develop other types of receptors that would cease to be sensitive to these ancient compounds, phylogenetically speaking. However, if we can learn anything from evolutionary biology, it is that everything is recycled. Evolution rarely works by creating entirely new protein structures, so the plant and animal kingdoms, including humans, share a large number of these structures. Simply put, if something works, why change it? Why devote energy to changing it? Let us remember again the difficulties plants faced in accessing basic resources. All forms of life that have ever existed on Earth, all except a small number of primates and domestic animals in the last few centuries, have suffered and agonized throughout their existence. Therefore, the maximum utilization and exploitation of "whatever resources are available," of what is at their disposal, has been a great driving force of evolution. If an organism couldn't make do with what it had, it succumbed. Period. But in addition to taking advantage of archaic structures, it is also worth mentioning that, due to the fact that the human organism is highly complex, by only having diversified or minimally altered these structures to form others, these small ancient molecules are now capable of binding with even more receptors than they originally did, because with increasing complexity the potential number of receptors to bind to increases exponentially.

Modifying Receptor Function

When a molecule binds to a receptor, it can modify its activity in certain ways. It is important to know what specific effects each substance has on receptor systems, as this is the beginning of a whole chain of effects that can be inferred with considerable certainty.

First, a substance can act as an *agonist*. Substances that activate the receptor "in its usual mode of operation" are called agonists. That is, an agonist is any substance that makes the receptor work in the same way as the chemicals that we have inside our body (endogenous) also make them work. There is only one slight nuance, and that is that agonist substances often activate the receptor more potently, compared to how potently endogenous substances activate it. For example, LSD activates serotonin receptors much more potently than serotonin itself. This, of course, does not happen in all cases. There are also agonists that activate the receptor with a potency similar to that of endogenous substances or even less potently. In that case they are called partial agonists, but we will not go into them in more detail.

We can also find substances that act as *antagonists*. As the word itself indicates, antagonist produces the opposite of an agonistic action. If agonists activate the receptor, go in their favor, antagonists deactivate it, they hinder their normal functioning. In a way, we can say that they block the receptor. There are several types of antagonists, but we will

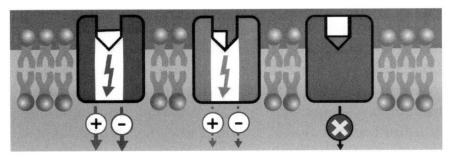

Figure 9. Representation of agonist ligands (the first receptor), partial agonists (the center receptor), and antagonists (the last receptor). While in the first and second there is receptor activation with variable potency, the receptors to which antagonistic ligands are bound remain blocked and have no effect. (See also color plate 2.)

see some of them in more detail later, including the implications of one type of antagonism or another.

Of course, there are many other ways to modify the functions of receptors. In addition to agonists and antagonists, there may be partial agonists, as we have seen, inverse agonists, or other types of interaction. However, agonism and antagonism are the basic interactions and the ones to remember first. Other interactions will be duly explained in each particular case.

WHY PSYCHEDELIC PHARMACOLOGY?

It is worth asking at this point why it is important to describe the pharmacology of psychedelic drugs. There are many reasons. The first is that these products have been used for centuries, even millennia, in different regions and cultures. They have been sacralized, institutionalized, and their users persecuted throughout history, always forming part of popular culture in one way or another. The truth is that, when we approach these substances, we immediately realize that they constitute a cultural phenomenon that transcends any simplistic and fragmented explanation that takes into account only part of the story. We feel that in order to begin to understand the fact that so many people throughout human history have decided to experiment with substances that profoundly transform their reality, anthropological texts are necessary, but also botanical, psychological, and theological texts. At the base of all these explanations is also the need to understand these substances from a pharmacological point of view, namely, why there are molecules that produce these particular effects and what makes them so special.

This first reason is perhaps rather ontological. We seek to understand the phenomenon at its best, integrating all its aspects and nuances. However, another reason may simply be the relevance that these substances have had for the development of disciplines such as pharmacology and psychopharmacology, since they have been more important than many would be willing to admit.

The importance of psychedelic drugs in these disciplines can be placed in two different historical moments. The first is in the mid-nineteenth century, where many authors place the birth of psychopharmacology due to the pioneering experiments and theoretical contributions of Moreau de Tours. This French psychiatrist used different plants and products with psychoactive properties (hashish, belladonna, ether, opium, or black henbane, among others) to study the human mind and mental disorders. In fact, he was the first to attribute mental illness to dysfunctions of the brain, which, according to Moreau de Tours, could be corrected using drugs, an idea that, at the time, was quite revolutionary.

A second historical moment, also crucial, occurs approximately a century later, between the 1940s and 1950s, when LSD is discovered by the Swiss chemist Albert Hofmann. The very obvious possibility of modifying mental functions with a chemical substance ended up securing the foundations of modern psychopharmacology, which were based on the certainty that our behavior and our thoughts were determined by internal chemicals and that, when they were altered (that is, when there was a mental disorder), it was as a consequence of an imbalance between said chemicals, and therefore possible to intervene to recover a healthy balance. The discovery of the psychoactive effects of LSD, but also the discovery of the first antipsychotic (chlorpromazine) and the effects of lithium salts on mood disorders, catapulted basic research in search of internal chemicals that would be related with the normal functioning of our brain and its disorders. A long-distance race ensued that would lead, a few years later, to the discovery and identification of serotonin and other neurotransmitters, with such monumental implications for research and understanding of brain functions that they are still being revealed today. The discoverers of serotonin, by the way, also conducted interaction studies between this substance and LSD, since they assumed that the powerful effects of LSD could have something to do with it. However, it was other groups, years later, who showed that serotonin was essential for the pharmacological action of LSD.

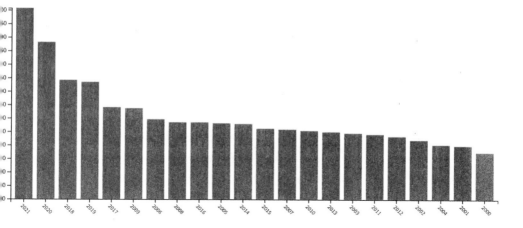

Figure 10. Number of scientific publications on psychedelic drugs
(on the vertical axis), classified by year (on the horizontal axis, starting from
2021 on the left and ranging to 2000 on the right).
Source: Web of Science. Graphic elaborated by the author.

Today, we are facing an unexpected and growing explosion of research on psychedelic drugs, as can be seen in figure 10. About ten years ago, the scientific activity around these drugs could be perfectly mapped and all the laboratories and research centers that carried out studies on these substances could be located. However, this is currently a very difficult, if not impossible, task, as many researchers in fields such as toxicology, anthropology, pharmacology, neuroscience, or psychology, who had never shown interest in these drugs before, are now turning en masse to investigating them.

PHARMACOLOGY AND COMPLEXITY

Whether for an ontological or historical reason, knowing the pharmacology of psychedelic drugs will allow us to delve into the mechanisms that underlie their mysterious effects. However, before embarking on the adventure, it is necessary to be a little cautious. Although here we expose the latest state-of-the-art knowledge at the pharmacological level to reveal the mechanisms of psychedelic drugs, these mechanisms will not provide us with an ultimate explanation of their effects.

For almost the entire modern history of science, a reductionist approach has been taken to explain complex phenomena. Reductionism is fine for a first, fragmentary level of analysis, as a way to start and not be overwhelmed by phenomena that are hard to grasp. It is also useful for explaining these phenomena in a pedagogical way, for students and laypeople alike to "get the picture" of something that would take too long to fully explain. However, reductionist views have often been confused with the much more complex reality they were trying to explain, leading us to believe that their "reduced" version of reality is the "real" one. In the case of psychedelics, this is a common occurrence. To the question "How do psychedelic drugs exert their effects?" the response is usually given "through the 5-HT2A receptor." But that does not explain anything; it does not answer the real question of "how." The fact that most psychedelics activate this receptor, and the fact that, if pharmacologically blocked, they no longer have an effect, does not explain the profound alteration of the state of consciousness that takes place.

Most of the basic processes carried out by the organism at a cellular and subcellular level can be explained by physical laws. Everything that happens at those levels, like diffusion, concentration gradient, and flow dynamics, is perfectly explainable in mathematical terms. The fact that it is explainable in mathematical terms and that we have a firm understanding of what is happening implies that we can predict it. Prediction is the basis of modern science; it is the pinnacle of the entire process of scientific inquiry. When you have the ability to predict something, it is because you have understood it perfectly, you have unraveled how it works, you have applied a law that is invariably fulfilled. It is the basis of deterministic models. When you predict, you literally "see" the future because you know what will happen if you modify certain elements of the phenomenon you are studying.

To focus this explanation on the human body, deterministic models in medicine have allowed substantial advancements in the knowledge of our body and in therapeutic methods to increase well-being and quality of life. Thus, applying basic knowledge of physics, we know that it is a good idea to prescribe a diuretic drug to a patient with hypertension because we know that the resistance to flow must be decreased to maintain an adequate pressure. If we reduce the volume of the blood (by excreting part of the water it contains, using a diuretic) we reduce the resistance to flow, so that the necessary force of the heart to pump blood will be less, thus reducing blood pressure. The same thing happens in the case of our brain. We can accurately describe how neurons communicate, how action potentials are produced, even how a certain neurotransmitter is released when we apply an exogenous molecule.

However, these basic principles of physics and associated deterministic models become meaningless in the face of complex systems and emergent properties. Even when we take an example like the above, regarding hypertension medication, although it is an elegant and simple model, we must not forget that we are not dealing with a closed system. We are not acting on a system of valves and currents that is not connected to anything else. We are acting on a highly complex system (the circulatory system) directly connected to other complex systems (immune, digestive), which in turn constitute an even more complex system (our body). This is why, even though we understand what happens at that micro-level of flow resistance when we administer a diuretic drug, we don't really know how much water the patient is losing. We do not know the exact volume of water that it is capable of losing, nor what volume would be ideal to lose. We also don't know what other effects the diuretic drug is having on the system. A known risk of diuretics is, in fact, the loss of potassium. When potassium levels are low, intracellular calcium levels in heart muscle cells increase, inducing an abnormal pattern of action potentials that may lead to the appearance of life-threatening arrhythmias. Deafness, both temporary and chronic, due to damage to the stria vascularis, is also a common risk associated with diuretic drugs.

When we study complex systems like the human body, even if we understand the basic mechanisms of their operation, we cannot apply deterministic models, because we cannot predict with certainty. We don't have that ability. Therefore, in medicine, when we carry out any intervention (such as prescribing a diuretic) we cannot know for sure if the drug will work, or if it will cause any of the side effects described in the literature. We move in a field of probabilities and not certainties. In the face of complex systems, uncertainty is the norm.

If we move with uncertainty with a hypertensive patient, imagine the case of human consciousness and its different states. We don't even need to go as far as human consciousness. With our understanding of physics and deterministic models, we cannot even explain higher functions such as language. They are emergent properties that are beyond the understanding of the particular elements that, after all, sustain them. That is to say, we can state that language is produced thanks to a certain neuronal activity, which we understand quite well, but we cannot explain language based on said neuronal activity. The same thing happens in the case of consciousness, as we said, although in this case we still don't even know with certainty what it is about. We know that it is there, we know that it is an "awareness," but since it is not a function that can be activated or deactivated (although perhaps psychedelics may help us in this) its study has been extraordinarily limited.

That is why we must emphasize that what is described in this book are the processes that underlie the effects of psychedelic drugs, but that we will not explain these effects. The impact of psychedelics on the psyche could only be explained if we had a complete and detailed map of the "black box" that currently exists between neuronal activity and the person's conscious (mental) sphere. Even if we did, we still could not apply the deterministic models mentioned above, because, just as each body reacts differently to a hypertensive drug, each mind also reacts differently to a psychedelic drug.

William Withering (1741–99, physician, geologist, chemist, and botanist) said that "remedies" are much more complex than the very diseases for which they are prescribed: "While the latter are in the hands of nature and similarities can always be drawn, the former are subject to the whims, inaccuracies and clumsiness of the human race." In the case of psychedelics, we are faced with a special type of complexity, since these are not only subject to the complexity of our body but also to that of our mind. The reader will find few assertions about the ultimate effects of psychedelic drugs in this book, but, another scholar, E. Duclaux, also said that science advances precisely because nothing is ever certain.[6]

REFERENCES FOR FURTHER STUDY

Hofmann A, Bouso JC. 2018. LSD: cómo descubrí el acido y lo que pasó después en el mundo [How I discovered acid and what happened next in the world]. Barcelona (Spain): Arpa Editions. Introduction, notes, and epilogue by José Carlos Bouso. Spanish.

López-Muñoz F, Álamo C. 2007. Historia de la psicofarmacología [History of psychopharmacology]. Volume 1. Madrid (Spain): Pan American Medical Publishing House. Spanish.

Ona G, Bouso JC. 2021. Towards the use of whole natural products in psychedelic research and therapy: synergy, multi-target profiles, and beyond [Monograph]. In Rahman A (editor), Frontiers in natural product chemistry. Bentham Science Publishers (location unknown).

Richards W. 2015. Sacred knowledge: psychedelics and religious experiences. New York (NY): Columbia University Press.

---

6. Born in 1840, Duclaux was a French mycologist, biologist, and chemist. Considered a leading intellectual of the time, he worked for most of his career as an assistant to Louis Pasteur.

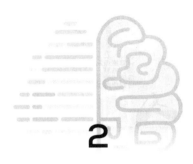

2

Pharmacological Classification of the Main Psychedelic Drugs

Structures and Major Groups

The human spirit advances continuously, but always in a spiral.

JOHANN W. GOETHE

In this chapter we will look at the main psychedelic drugs that will be discussed in the rest of the book. At the same time, we will classify them as rigorously as we know how so that, from the outset, the different groups that exist are clear to us. However, it must be said that there are many different ways of classifying psychedelic drugs, either according to their effects, their pharmacological properties, or their contexts of use. Therefore, the classification that is presented below should not be understood as canonical, but simply as one more classification of all the options available until now.

Psychedelic drugs can be classified into six basic categories: simple tryptamines, ergolamines, phenethylamines, NMDA receptor antagonists, new tryptamines, and atypical psychedelics. Let's look at each of these groups in detail.

SIMPLE TRYPTAMINES, INCLUDING PSILOCYBIN AND DMT

This group is called simple tryptamines because even though there are tryptamines in other groups too, they show some differences in their molecular structure. Tryptamines, as the word indicates, are molecules derived from tryptophan, an essential amino acid for our organism, present both in our body and in our diet. Some neurotransmitters are formed from tryptophan, such as serotonin, but also some molecules with psychoactive properties.

TABLE I. MAIN SIMPLE TRYPTAMINES AND THEIR FULL NAMES

Simple tryptamines	Full name
Bufotenin	5-hydroxy-N,N-dimethyltryptamine
DMT	N,N-dimethyltryptamine
5-MeO-DMT	5-methoxy-N,N-dimethyltryptamine
Psilocybin	4-phosphoryloxy-N,N-dimethyltryptamine
Psilocin	4-hydroxy-N,N-dimethyltryptamine

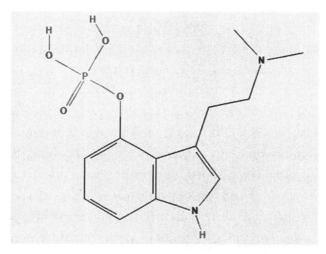

Figure 11. Psilocybin molecule.

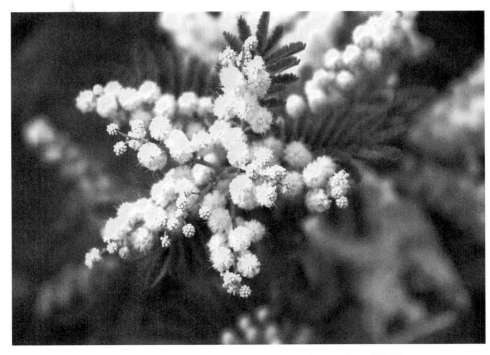

Figure 12. *Acacia dealbata* (Mimosa), plant rich in DMT.
(See also color plate 3.)

Within the group of simple tryptamines we can find psilocybin, the active principle of the fungi of the genus *Psilocybe*, or N,N-dimethyltryptamine (DMT). Psilocybin is a prodrug, which means that it is an inactive substance that when ingested is metabolized into another substance that is pharmacologically active (in this case psilocin). Other examples of prodrugs are levodopa (metabolizes into dopamine), diazepam (metabolizes into oxazepam), or aspirin (metabolizes into salicylic acid). DMT is naturally produced in our body, fulfilling unknown functions at the moment, and can be found in the same way in many mammals and in a high percentage of plants (of the genus *Mimosa*, for example) and trees (citrus, such as lemon and orange trees, and of the genus *Acacia*). It must be said that these tryptamines are highly safe from a toxicological point of view, the risk of overdose being highly unlikely.

ERGOLAMINES, INCLUDING LSD

As their name also indicates, these are a group of substances derived from ergot, the fungus *Claviceps purpurea* (as well as others of the genus *Claviceps*) that colonizes cereals and other grasses and has psychoactive properties. However, the consumption of *C. purpurea* leads to some serious health problems. For example, given its powerful vasoconstrictor action, it can cause gangrene in the upper and lower limbs. As this fungus colonizes cereals, in the Middle Ages its accidental consumption in the form of flour or bread was the cause of numerous outbreaks of poisoning with the fungus, which were popularly referred to as the "fire of San Antonio." Some species of the genus *Claviceps* (like the *C. paspali*) can be eaten raw, without risk of losing a few fingers in the process, to achieve its psychoactive effects.

What many species of this genus have in common is the presence of ergine (LSA, also present in plants such as *Ipomoea violacea* and responsible for its psychoactive effects) or ergotamine, among other substances. From ergotamine it is possible to synthesize LSD, or lysergic acid diethylamide, one of the most acclaimed and equally reviled psychedelics. Like the simple tryptamines, LSD is also very safe for our

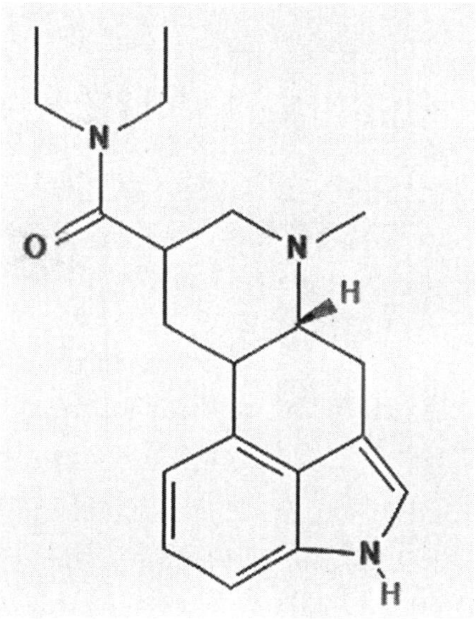

Figure 13. LSD molecule.

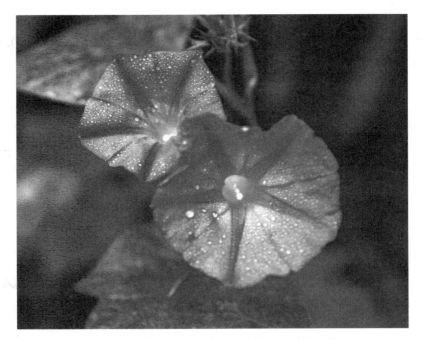

Figure 14. *Ipomoea violacea* (Morning Glory),
with seeds containing LSA. (See also color plate 4.)

body. A recent case report described a woman who mistook LSD for cocaine and snorted approximately 55 mg of LSD, some 550 times more than the usual 100 microgram dose. The effects lasted several days, with repeated vomiting especially during the first twelve hours, but she experienced no physical problems or signs of serious intoxication. In fact, a nagging pain she had been suffering for years disappeared for a few days, so she stopped using morphine (prescribed for that pain) for five days, without experiencing withdrawal symptoms.

PHENETHYLAMINES, INCLUDING MESCALINE AND MDMA

This second group includes substances that do not have a tryptamine nucleus, and therefore are not derived from tryptophan, but from phenylalanine, another essential amino acid. Among the substances in this group we find mescaline, an active principle of cacti such as peyote (*Lophophora williamsii*), San Pedro (*Echinopsis pachanoi*), or MDMA, also known as ecstasy. The latter also has a strong structural similarity to amphetamines, so it really belongs in an indeterminate space. Due to its molecular structure, it is somewhat more stimulating and does not produce as dramatic effects on perception as other psychedelics, but it is often defined as "empathogenic" due to its ability to generate closeness and feelings of affability toward other people.

TABLE 2. MAIN SUBSTANCES INCLUDED IN THE PHENETHYLAMINES GROUP AND THEIR FULL NAMES

Phenethylamines	Full name
Mescaline	3,4,5-trimethoxyphenethylamine
MDA	3,4-methylenedioxyamphetamine
MDMA	3,4-methylenedioxymethamphetamine
2-CB	4-bromo-2,5-dimethoxyphenethylamine

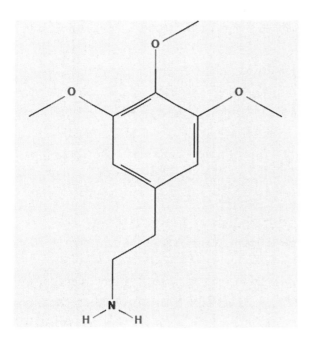

Figure 15. Mescaline molecule.

NMDA RECEPTOR ANTAGONISTS,
INCLUDING KETAMINE

NMDA receptors (N-methyl-D-aspartic acid) are a type of glutamate receptor. Glutamate is an amino acid that can be defined as the "fuel" of neurons. Substances that act as antagonists to this receptor tend to produce psychoactive effects that are also very characteristic. For example, ketamine is an NMDA receptor antagonist, and its effects are defined as dissociative, in the sense that one can have the feeling of being disconnected from their environment or from oneself, leading to out-of-body experiences. A curiosity about ketamine: it was recently discovered that the fungus *Pochonia chlamydosporia* produces ketamine with the intention of combating certain pathogens.[1] Apparently, ketamine would have a very interesting antihelminthic effect. There are other fascinating examples of molecules that were first synthesized in the laboratory and years later were identified in nature. It seems that ketamine is one of these cases, so from now on we can consider ketamine as a natural substance.

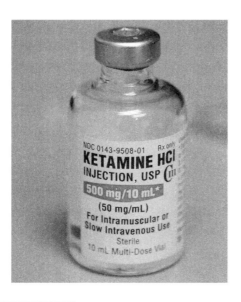

Figure 16. Ketamine bottle.

---

1. Ferreira SR, Machado ART, Furtado LF, et al. 2020. Ketamine can be produced by *Pochonia chlamydosporia*: an old molecule and a new anthelmintic? Parasites & Vectors 13(527).

A substance similar to ketamine is PCP or phencyclidine, popularly known as "angel dust." PCP was marketed as a general anesthetic for a few years, until cases were reported of patients recently released from the operating room presenting symptoms of psychosis, which led to the belief that perhaps an alternative ought to be sought. Another NMDA receptor antagonist is dextromethorphan (a cough suppressant). At high doses it produces hallucinations and other psychedelic-like symptoms, although it is actually an opioid, so not everyone would agree to include it on this list.

NEW TRYPTAMINES

Since the chemical creativity of the Shulgins,[2] hundreds of new molecules with psychedelic effects have been created. They can be called "new mines," "legal highs," or "new psychoactive substances," but all of them share the characteristic of being derived from other drugs and, in most cases, not being controlled, since they are "new" substances. We put "new" in quotation marks because, although many of them were actually synthesized forty or fifty years ago, they only recently began to circulate in informal markets.

In this group we find substances such as 5-MeO-DIPT, 5-MeO-AMT, and 4-OH-MET. These substances tend to be considered more dangerous than the psychedelics of the simple tryptamine group or other groups; however, their most dangerous aspect is the lack of information that surrounds them. Since no animal or human studies have been conducted, because they do not have a long tradition of use like LSD, or history like *Psilocybe* mushrooms, their properties or safety profile are often unknown.

---

2. Ann and Alexander Shulgin (therapist and chemist, respectively) have gone down in history for their activity related to the synthesis of many drugs and the dissemination of information on their possible therapeutic effects. Both are authors of the books *PiHKAL: A Chemical Love Story* and *TiHKAL: The Continuation*, their most outstanding works. Alexander passed away in 2014 and Ann passed away in 2022.

ATYPICAL PSYCHEDELICS

In this section we will talk about three psychoactive plants: *Tabernanthe iboga*, *Salvia divinorum*, and *Datura stramonium*. All three have been used for at least several centuries and have been part of traditional medicine and the therapeutic arsenal of different cultures. Let's see them in detail.

Tabernanthe iboga

T. iboga is a plant native to the African continent, specifically Central West Africa. There is a long tradition of its use by the Pygmies and other peoples of the Congo and Gabon, mainly. This plant contains many alkaloids and compounds with a unique structure. The best known of these is ibogaine, which is found in high concentrations in the root bark. This molecule has antiaddictive properties that are often described as "magical" and is capable of considerably reducing the *craving* (or compulsive use), such as the withdrawal syndrome, produced by different drugs of abuse, although it seems that ibogaine is especially effective in the treatment of opiate dependence, such as heroin or methadone.

Ibogaine is capable of modulating different receptor systems and other biological targets that we will see in the next chapter, although that is not why it is classified as an "atypical" psychedelic, since other substances also modulate different receptors. This denomination is rather due to the fact that it produces psychoactive effects through other mechanisms not directly related to serotonin receptors. Unlike most tryptamines, ibogaine is also cardiotoxic, so there is a death risk at doses not much higher than those usually used in therapeutic settings.

Salvia divinorum

Originally from Mexico, this plant of the mint family has been widely used in traditional Mazatec medicine for different purposes both medicinal and spiritual. Its active ingredient is salvinorin-A, which also

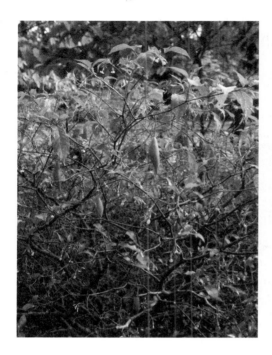

Figure 17. *Tabernanthe iboga* (Iboga), plant containing ibogaine. (See also color plate 5.)

has a rather peculiar molecular structure. It is a potent kappa-opioid receptor agonist, with apparently no action to any other opioid receptors (which is quite rare). But, in addition, it was also the first known agonist of these receptors that did not have a nitrogen nucleus, which may play an important role in its characteristic effect on the receptor. We will see this in more detail in the next chapter.

Salvinorin-A is also characterized by a high level of frustration among many of its users, as it is somewhat difficult to administer effectively. When the leaves of the plant are used, the traditional method is to chew a certain number of leaves (depending on the intention) until the user can access other states of consciousness. Recreational users who resort to this route, even chewing large amounts of leaves, find it difficult to report intense experiences, beyond a slight "high" or dizziness. Another way to consume salvinorin-A is through "standardized" products, in theory consisting of ground leaves enriched with pure salvinorin-A at different concentrations. This seldom goes beyond just theory and marketing strategies, as some studies have found no

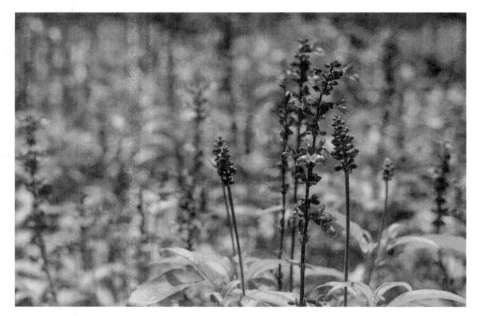

Figure 18. *Salvia divinorum* (Salvia), plant rich in salvinorin-A.
(See also color plate 6.)

significant differences in the content of salvinorin-A between products with labels reporting different "potencies."

An alternative consumption strategy is the acquisition of pure salvinorin-A, something that does not seem to be very frequent in informal markets and is mainly used in clinical trials, such as the one mentioned above, in which this author participated. In cases where high doses of the pure substance have been used, reported subjective experiences have been little short of spooky, something that also differs from the typical psychedelic experiences. In the case of salvinorin-A, it is usual for the person to feel that they are entering a reality that is "more real" than their usual reality. Experiences related to dimensionality modifications are also reported. Suddenly the person can appear in a two-dimensional space, or in a multidimensional one. It may also seem to them that their whole body has been crushed on the ground and that a horde of dwarfs with shovels is coming to pick them up (real experience). It is also common to meet monsters or other beings, such as giants, gods, or alien creatures.

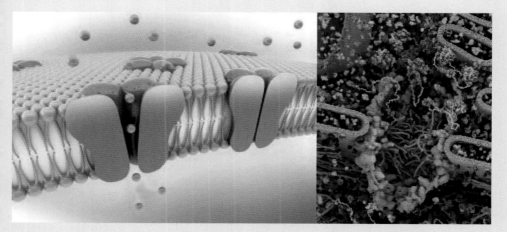

Plate 1. Graphic representation of brain receptors (*left*) and a real image of a receptor (*right*).

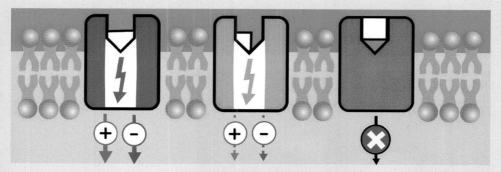

Plate 2. Representation of agonist ligands (the first receptor), partial agonists (the center receptor), and antagonists (the last receptor). While in the first and second there is receptor activation with variable potency, the receptors to which antagonistic ligands are bound remain blocked and have no effect.

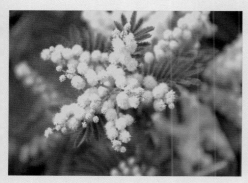

Plate 3. *Acacia dealbata* (Mimosa), plant rich in DMT.

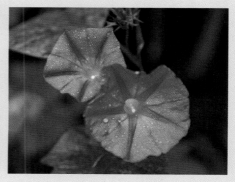

Plate 4. *Ipomoea violacea* (Morning Glory), with seeds containing LSA.

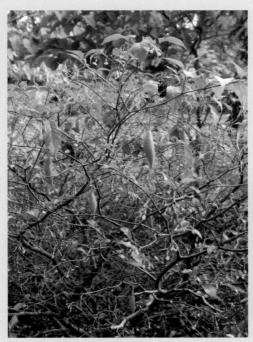

Plate 5. *Tabernanthe iboga* (Iboga), plant containing ibogaine.

Plate 6. *Salvia divinorum* (Salvia), plant rich in salvinorin-A.

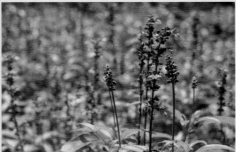

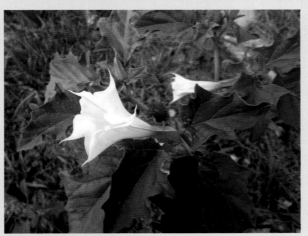

Plate 7. *Datura stramonium* (Jimsonweed), plant rich in tropane alkaloids.

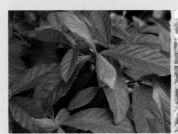 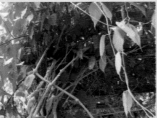 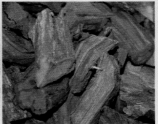

Plate 8. *Mimosa hostilis* (*left* image) and *Banisteriopsis caapi* (*center* and *right* images), plants used for ayahuasca decocting. For full source information, see page 86.

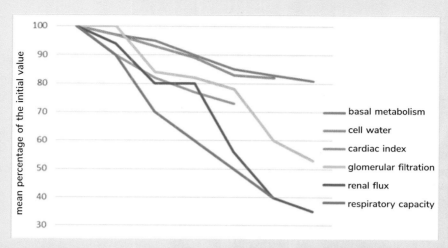

Plate 9. Modification of physiological parameters with age. On the vertical axis, mean percentage of the initial value, and on the horizontal axis, age.

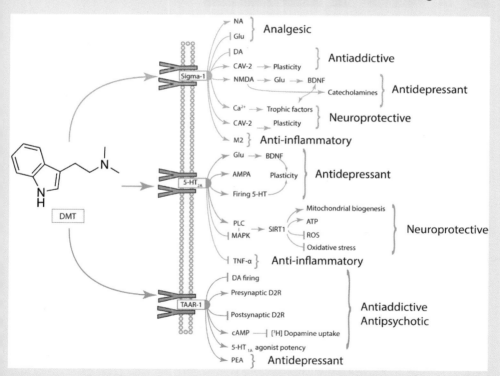

Plate 10. Main mechanisms of action by which DMT exerts analgesic, antiaddictive, antidepressant, neuroprotective, anti-inflammatory, and antipsychotic effects. Original image from the article: Ona G, Bouso JC. 2021. Therapeutic potential of natural psychoactive drugs for central nervous system disorders: a perspective from polypharmacology. Current Medicinal Chemistry 28(1):53–68. Reproduced with the authors' permission.

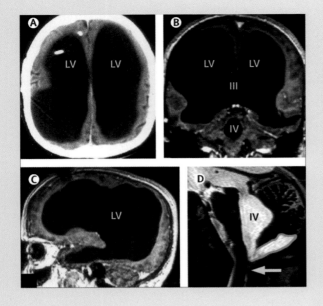

Plate 11. Brain images of a patient who, despite having only 25 percent of his brain mass, led a completely normal life. Original image from the article: Feuillet L, Dufour H. 2007. Brain of a white-collar worker. The Lancet 370(9583):262. Reproduced with the authors' permission.

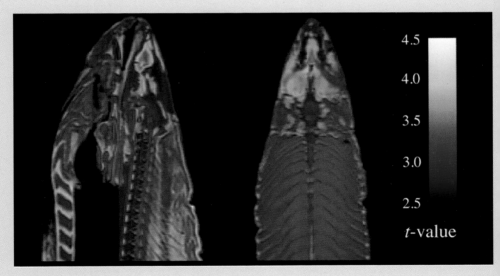

Plate 12. Brain activity reported by magnetic resonance imaging in a specimen of *Salmo salar* (salmon), while being shown images of individuals of the *Homo sapiens* species interacting. Original image from the article: Bennett CM, Wolford GL, Miller MB. 2009. The principled control of false positives in neuroimaging. Social Cognitive and Affective Neuroscience 4(4):417–422. Reproduced with the authors' permission.

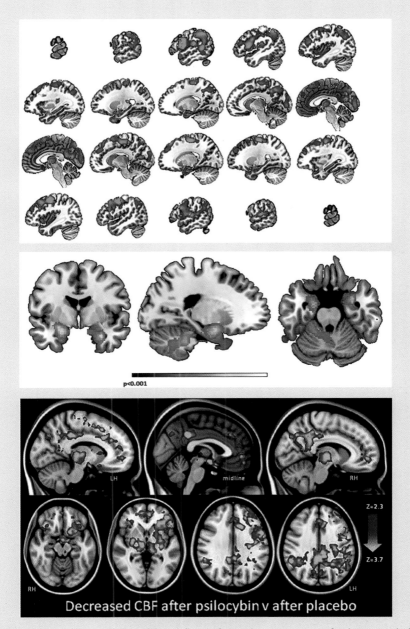

Decreased CBF after psilocybin v after placebo

Plate 13. Variations in cerebral blood flow after administration of salvinorin-A (*top*) and psilocybin (*bottom*). In the case of salvinorin-A, extensive decreases in blood flow were reported in the cortex of all cerebral lobes (frontal, temporal, medial, and occipital) and increases in flow in subcortical regions, mainly the amygdala, hippocampus, and cerebellum. Psilocybin, by contrast, only showed more discreet decreases in blood flow in some regions of the cortex and in subcortical regions, such as the thalamus. No flux increase was observed in this case. All images reproduced with the authors' permission. For full source information, see page 122.

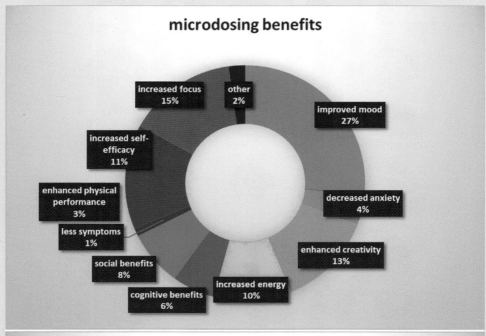

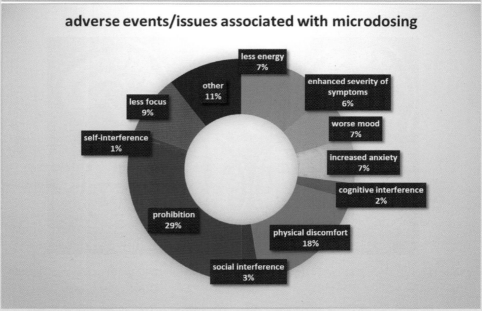

Plate 14. The image has been adapted and translated from the article: Anderson T, Petranker R, Christopher A, Rosenbaum D, Weissman C, Dinh-Williams L-A, Hui K, Hapke E. 2019. Psychedelic microdosing benefits and challenges: an empirical codebook. *Harm Reduction Journal* 16:43.

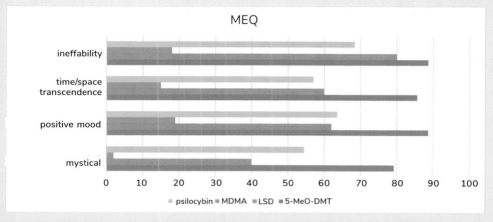

Plate 15. MEQ (Mystical Experiences Questionnaire) scores after the administration of psilocybin, MDMA, LSD, and 5-MeO-DMT in clinical trial settings. Chart prepared by the author.

Plate 16. APZ (Altered States of Consciousness) questionnaire scores after administration of salvinorin-A, psilocybin, MDE, DMT, and ayahuasca in clinical trial settings. Chart prepared by the author.

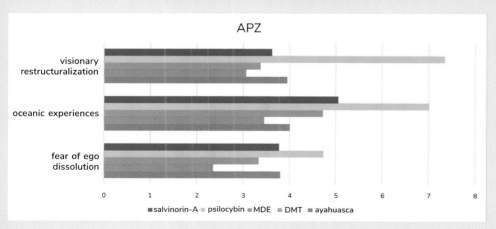

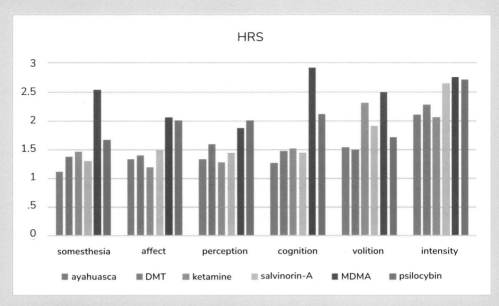

Plate 17. HRS (Hallucinogen Rating Scale) questionnaire scores after administration of ayahuasca, DMT, ketamine, salvinorin-A, MDMA, and psilocybin in clinical trial settings. Chart prepared by the author.

Plate 18. The 5D-ASC (Five Dimensional-Altered States of Consciousness) questionnaire scores after administration of ibogaine, ketamine, MDMA, psilocybin, and LSD in clinical trial settings. Chart prepared by the author.

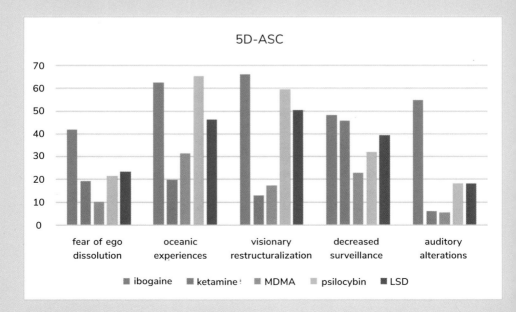

All of these experiences are quite idiosyncratic to salvinorin-A and most closely resemble the idea of psychedelic hallucinations typical of the social imagery, which are actually the exception to the norm.

Datura stramonium

This plant has been used for millennia in both Eastern and European regions. In European history it is known, above all, for having been part of the therapeutic arsenal of healers. Its effects are also associated with the archetypal image of the witch flying on a broom. (It has been hypothesized that *D. stramonium* ointments could have been smeared on the broomstick and that these, being absorbed by the vaginal mucosa, would have made women think they were flying when they felt their hallucinatory effects. And although humans are free to act as they see fit, and we cannot rule out any possibilities, the veracity of such accounts is disputed.)

D. stramonium should in fact be classified in a broader context, in the Solanaceae group, with plants such as black henbane (*Hyoscyamus niger*) or floripondio (*Brugmansia arborea*), all of them psychoactive and widely used in various rituals and medical practices. It is important to note that not all plants belonging to this family are psychoactive, since tomatoes or potatoes are also Solanaceae. However, it is worth remembering that there are various plants belonging to this family that are, and moreover, that they are because they contain similar components.

D. stramonium and other psychoactive Solanaceae are rich in tropane alkaloids, that is, they contain a tropane nucleus, just as others contain a tryptophan nucleus. The concentrations of these alkaloids vary according to the plant or the habitat, but in the case of the *D. stramonium* we found a high concentration of atropine, hyoscyamine, and scopolamine. Atropine has been used for more than a century, and is still used today, as a cardiotonic. For example, when the heart rate is below forty or fifty beats per minute and there is a cardiac risk, atropine is administered to raise the number of beats. It is also used in ophthalmology to dilate the pupils. If you have ever been to the eye doctor and were given a few drops to dilate your pupils, it was atropine. Hyoscyamine also has a long history of use in Western medicine, primarily to treat gastrointestinal disorders. Scopolamine is also currently used, especially in surgery, to reduce salivation and respiratory secretions.

Although the therapeutic doses of these compounds are not psychoactive, when consumed at higher doses they induce severe intoxications, with the presence of hallucinations, confusion, delusions, blurred vision, tachycardia, or dehydration. In the worst cases, the person can also lose consciousness and go into a coma. The effects, depending on the dose, can last more than twenty-four hours and, in general, intoxicated people do not remember the experience. Due to this last characteristic, it has been suggested that some tropane alkaloids, especially scopolamine, may be used by sexual assailants and rapists. These preparations have been popularly called "burundanga." Although it cannot be ruled out that in some cases it has been used for these purposes, it should be noted that the drug most used to manipulate the will of people, and erase the memories of what happened, is alcohol.

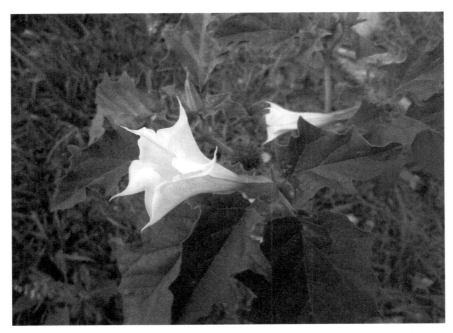

Figure 19. *Datura stramonium* (Jimsonweed), plant rich in tropane alkaloids.
(See also color plate 7.)

REFERENCES FOR FURTHER STUDY

Kelmendi B, Kaye AP, Pittenger C, Kwan AC. 2022. Psychedelics. Current Biology 32(2):R63–R67.

Nichols D, Johnson MW, Nichols CD. 2017. Psychedelics as medicines: an emerging new paradigm. Clinical Pharmacology & Therapeutics 101(2):209–219.

Nichols D. 2016. Psychedelics. Pharmacological Reviews 68(2):264–355.

Psycheplants. 2018. Información sobre plantas psicoactivas [Information about psychoactive plants]. Barcelona (Spain): ICEERS Foundation. Spanish.

Waters K. 2021. Pharmacologic similarities and differences among hallucinogens. The Journal of Clinical Pharmacology 61(S2):100–113.

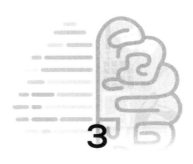

3

Biological Targets of Psychedelic Drugs

*If we can wake up when we dream, when we are awake,
can we wake up even more?*

ANONYMOUS

When a psychedelic drug is used, as is the case with any other substance, its active ingredients bind to a series of biological targets. We are going to talk mainly about receptors, as they are the main targets, although it is important to remember that these are not the only binding sites, in pharmacological terms. Drugs, in general, can also act on enzymes, transporters, and many other targets. However, this is a deeper and more complex level of analysis, mainly used for very detailed investigations that do not necessarily concern the final effects of the substances in question. For this reason, in this chapter, we will limit ourselves to describing the effects at the receptor level.

"Receptor" is a concept that was first cited in a publication from 1900, by Paul Ehrlich, a German scientist who made great contributions in the field of therapeutics and bacteriology. Although, at that time, it was thought that receptors were selective only for certain toxins, today we know that they fulfill elementary functions, being essential for intercellular communication or the regulation of practically all the functions of our body. Receptors are generally found in the cell membrane, although they can also be located at the intracellular or intranuclear level. When a molecule (or ligand) binds to a receptor, the effects that occur will depend on various factors, including the characteristics of the ligand itself, the type of binding that is established, the complexes that the receptor has formed with other receptors, or the tissues where the receptor is found, among others.

With this in mind, we have to understand phrases such as "this drug is an agonist of the X receptor, therefore it has a Y effect," which we have all heard or read at some point, as a very reductive statement that can only be applied to the specific ligand being observed, and can never be applied to other ligands with agonistic effects of the X receptor. Let's see an example. LSD primarily exerts its action through its agonist effect on the 5-HT2A receptor, a particular type of serotonin receptor. Lisuride, a medication also derived from ergot, is a 5-HT2A agonist, which binds to this receptor in much the same way as LSD. However, lisuride does not produce any relevant psychoactive effects. Thus we see that the fact that it binds to the same receptors as LSD does not guarantee that it will produce the same effect. We have to keep this in mind when we talk about both psychedelic drugs and drugs in general.

Another additional point is that most of the substances we are going to discuss here bind to many different receptors. And this might be why they are especially safe from a toxicological standpoint. Other hallucinogenic substances, like 25I-NBOMe, act as a highly potent and selective full agonist of the 5-HT2A receptor, and perhaps this is partly why they are more toxic. This is a hypothesis of mine, but there is some anecdotal evidence suggesting that throughout the research pipeline of new commercialized drugs, there is a kind of "natural selection" that allows those more promiscuous molecules, which affect more receptors, to reach the final stages of development, while those more selective toward specific receptors are discarded due to safety concerns. This fact might be related to the usual functioning of our organism, designed and prepared to modulate in a widely complex and robust way, ingesting and processing nutrients with multiple effects, leveraging enzymes for a multitude of different functions, and so on. In reality, such selective substances are a rarity in nature and our body might not be accustomed to dealing with them. There are exceptions to this as well. Salvinorin-A is very selective for a specific receptor but does not seem to be toxic. Although salvinorin-A seems to come from another universe and the rules and laws of our reality might not apply to it.

SIMPLE TRYPTAMINE TARGETS

The receptor primarily responsible for the psychoactive effects of simple tryptamines, as well as most of the groups we will discuss in this chapter, is the serotonin 5-HT2A receptor. Serotonin receptors, or 5-HT, are part of a large family of receptors called "G protein-coupled receptors" (GPCRs). GPCRs represent the main targets of any pharmacological substance (including those with psychoactive properties), since up to a third of all known substances will bind to these GPCRs. In the case of serotonin receptors, a general type of receptor (5-HT) and dozens of subtypes (5-HT1A, 5-HT1B, 5-HT1D, 5-HT2A, 5-HT2B, 5-HT2C, and so on) have been identified.

Several decades after the discovery of serotonin and its respective receptors, it was concluded that a specific subtype of these receptors (5-HT2A) was crucial for the psychoactive tryptamines to deploy their psychological effects. Some animal studies already suggested this idea in the 1970s and 1980s, but the definitive experiment came at the hands of the Franz X. Vollenweider team, in Switzerland, with a publication that appeared in the year 1998.[1] In this study, subjects were administered a 5-HT2A receptor antagonist drug (ketanserin) one and a half hours before they were given a dose of 0.25 mg per kilogram of body weight of psilocybin. They observed that the ketanserin effectively blocked the effects of the psilocybin, providing irre-

1. Vollenweider FX, Vollenweider-Scherpenhuyzen MFI, Babler A, Vogel H, Hell D. 1998. Psilocybin induces schizophrenia-like psychosis in humans via a serotonin-2 agonist action. NeuroReport 9, 3897–3902.

futable evidence of the decisive role that this receptor subtype plays in the psychoactive effects of psilocybin. A similar study was also carried out, years later, regarding ayahuasca. In this case the study was carried out by the Human Neuropsychopharmacology group of the Hospital de la Santa Creu i Sant Pau, in Barcelona, led by Dr. Jordi Riba. This study also confirmed that ketanserin could block the psychoactive effects of ayahuasca and thus of DMT, another simple tryptamine.

Although it is the 5-HT2A receptor that allows the psychoactive effects of tryptamines to unfold, this does not mean that the activation of this receptor is solely responsible for all of these effects. We can think of psychoactive effects as a series of domino pieces that fall one after another. The first of these pieces would be the 5-HT2A receptor, and this one, by "falling," would cause the fall of many others. In this successive fall of other "pieces," the first that we can mention is the beginning and propagation of action potentials in neurons containing 5-HT2A receptors (distributed throughout the cerebral cortex and subcortical brain regions, such as the amygdala or the hypothalamus). Therefore, we can say that the circulation of tryptamines, like psilocybin, cause activation of 5-HT2A receptors, which leads to increased depolarization of the neurons where these receptors are found, generating more action potentials and, therefore, resulting in an "excitability" effect, in general.

It is important to point out that this excited state does not mean we will find a greater general activation of all associated neurons and brain regions, since inhibitory neurons can also be excited and, therefore, result in remarkable decreases in activity. We can find an example of what the consequences of this extensive activation of 5-HT2A receptors may be in the neurons responsible for glutamate neurotransmission. This activation of 5-HT2A receptors induces a higher release of serotonin. When serotonin comes into contact with glutamatergic neurons, it dramatically increases the frequency with which they are depolarized (which means they are activated, as we have seen previously), especially those found in the frontal cortex. This greater activation of neurons by glutamate has been associated precisely with the effects related to the increase in neuroplasticity induced by different psychedelic drugs. We will delve deeper into this concept in the chapter on pharmacokinetics and pharmacodynamics.

Psilocybin

Psilocybin is the most representative (because it is the most studied) molecule of the group of simple tryptamines and may help us describe the general receptor binding profile in more detail. First, we will talk about psilocybin in particular, although it is worth mentioning that this is only one of the molecules that are found within a complex of chemical substances that are part of the mushrooms of the genus *Psilocybe*, the species *Psilocybe cubensis* being among the best known. Like any natural product, *P. cubensis* constitutes an entity with a highly complex phytochemical profile.[2]

> The most common feature in natural products is that we find in each of them tens, hundreds, or even thousands of different substances, which will have a highly complex effect when interacting with our body and with each other.

If describing the effects that a single molecule produces in our body is difficult, imagine what happens when we ingest hundreds of them. Although not all of them are biologically active, in other words, not producing a specific effect, even these are relevant when explaining the general effect of these natural products, since they will often *facilitate* or *hinder* the effects of other molecules that are active.[3]

It would be foolish not to dedicate some lines to other compounds

2. "Phytochemical profile" refers to the components that a given natural product contains. We know the phytochemical profile of a product when we are able to list all these components.
3. Readers who may be interested in delving into the pharmacology of natural products in general, but also of natural products with psychoactive effects, can consult Ona and Bouso (2021) (see full reference above at the end of chapter 1).

present in this genus of fungi, since, although the majority if not all research focuses on the use of isolated psilocybin, at the population level, the vast majority of people use mushrooms, which contain psilocybin, of course, but also many other substances. In this sense, we must proceed with some caution when reading the results of clinical or neuroscientific studies that have used psilocybin, since these findings may not explain all the effects experienced by users of psilocybin mushrooms, because, from a pharmacological point of view, we are talking about different products. Even many scientists refer to *Psilocybe* mushrooms simply as "psilocybin," reducing these complex fungi to a single substance. This approach overlooks the multitude of other compounds present and their pharmacological intricacies, as well as disregards the ancestral knowledge rooted in the use of the entire mushroom. Just as we do not define lemons solely by their vitamin C content, or coffee merely by its caffeine, we should not oversimplify *Psilocybe* mushrooms.

As we have previously described, the main pharmacological target that is largely relevant to explaining the complex effects of psilocybin (or rather, the psilocin; remember that psilocybin is a prodrug) is the 5-HT2A receptor. The targets that we will discuss now are those to which psilocin binds when it crosses the blood-brain barrier, accessing the brain. However, and although it may seem surprising, this is not its main target, pharmacologically speaking. The receptors that psilocin shows the highest affinity for are 5-HT1D, 5-HT2C, 5-HT2B, 5-HT5, 5-HT6, and 5-HT7, and, to a somewhat lesser degree, 5-HT1A (as can be seen, all serotonin receptors), showing a moderate affinity, clearly at a second level, for the 5-HT2A receptor. Although the affinity for the 5-HT2A receptor is not very high, it does continue to be essential for the deployment of psychoactive effects, because when specific antagonists of the 5-HT2A receptor are administered, thus preventing its binding to psilocin, the substance's effects are totally blocked, as was observed in the pioneering study by Vollenweider (1998) mentioned above.

The widespread affinity for so many serotonin subreceptors is a well-known phenomenon in pharmacology. In fact, it is to some extent expected that a ligand that binds to one receptor subtype, be it serotonin, dopamine, or any other receptor system, would also show affinity for other subtypes of that receptor. In reality, the relevance that this widespread binding profile may have for the psychoactive effects of psilocybin is unknown, although it is usually considered that these binding patterns are the ones that end up configuring the subjective particularities of each substance. This is due to the fact that even if non-5-HT2A receptors are not related to the induction of psychoactive effects, it does seem likely that they could "modulate" it to a certain extent. This is still the subject of intense debate, since it is also true that each experience, even in the same subject, is different and characteristic; therefore, it would be difficult to find an always stable and identifiable pattern of subjective effects associated with *P. cubensis* (not to mention the variability in the phytochemical profile of different samples of this species, which would also have repercussions in the variations of said effects). To finish with serotonin receptors, it remains to be noted that the 5-HT1A receptor is the main inhibitory receptor for serotonin. Following what we stated above, this means that the activation of this receptor by the psilocin will induce decreases in activity in certain regions or reductions in the release of other neurotransmitters, which in fact has been observed in some studies.[4,5]

Other receptors for which psilocin has also shown affinity are the histamine H1 receptors, the adrenergic alpha-2A and alpha-2B and dopamine D3 receptors. It is capable of inhibiting the serotonin transporter (SERT). The SERT is responsible for "picking up" part of the serotonin molecules found in the synaptic cleft (the space between the end of one neuron and the beginning of another), so its inhibition translates into higher concentrations of serotonin. As for the rest of the receptors, it seems that the role they can play in the psychoactive effects is irrelevant.

4. Mason NL, Kuypers K, Müller F, Reckweg J, Tse D, Toennes SW, Hutten N, Jansen J, Stiers P, Feilding A, Ramaekers JG. 2020. Me, myself, bye: regional alterations in glutamate and the experience of ego dissolution with psilocybin. Neuropsychopharmacology 45(12):2003–2011.
5. Lewis CR, Preller KH, Kraehenmann R, Michels L, Staempfli P, Vollenweider FX. 2017. Two dose investigation of the 5-HT-agonist psilocybin on relative and global cerebral blood flow. NeuroImage 159:70–78.

Only one dopamine receptor subtype (D2) has been associated with hallucinatory effects, but the dopamine receptor to which the psilocin binds (D3) seems not to be taking action in that regard. In fact, in some studies, specific D2 receptor antagonists have been administered together with psilocybin, observing that psychedelic effects were not blocked.

Apart from psilocin, other substances have been identified in the mushrooms of the genus *Psilocybe* that are capable of inhibiting monoamine oxidase (MAO), an enzyme responsible for degrading substances such as serotonin or dopamine, but also psilocin. In fact, MAO inhibitors play a crucial role in the case of ayahuasca, as we will see later. Therefore, the presence of these MAO-inhibiting molecules in the same mushroom can cause psilocybin to display a much greater effect and, in line with what has been commented on above, cause differences with respect to the profile of psychoactive effects described when mushrooms are consumed compared to when synthetic psilocybin is consumed, although the dose is the same in both cases.

TABLE 3. MAIN TARGETS OF PSILOCYBIN*

Psilocybin Targets	Ki
Serotonin receptors	
5-HT$_{1A}$	567.4
5-HT$_{1B}$	219.6
5-HT$_{1D}$	36.4
5-HT$_{2C}$	97.3
5-HT$_{2B}$	4.6
5-HT$_5$	83.7
5-HT$_6$	57
5-HT$_7$	3.5
5-HT$_{2A}$	107.2
SERT	3,801

*Ki is the inhibition constant, a parameter used to assess receptor affinity. The smaller the value of Ki, the greater the affinity.

TABLE 3. MAIN TARGETS OF PSILOCYBIN* (cont.)

Psilocybin Targets	Ki
Histamine receptors	
HI	304.6
Adrenergic receptors	
alpha$_{2A}$	1,379
alpha$_{2B}$	1,894
Dopamine receptors	
D$_2$	>10,000
D$_3$	2,645

*Ki is the inhibition constant, a parameter used to assess receptor affinity. The smaller the value of Ki, the greater the affinity.

DMT and Ayahuasca

DMT is another simple tryptamine that shows a binding profile to receptors somewhat differently than psilocin. This molecule is taken isolated and purified, inhaling the vapors that result from its combustion, although it is also found in ayahuasca, an original infusion from the Amazon jungle, increasingly known in our contemporary societies. Due to the clear expansion of its consumption, we will also dedicate a few lines to explain this drink's complex binding to receptors.

When pure, isolated DMT enters the bloodstream, it mainly activates 5-HT1A, 5-HT2A, and 5-HT2C receptors. It also acts as an agonist in a receptor that is very interesting from a therapeutic point of view, the sigma-1. This receptor is widely distributed throughout the CNS, heart, liver, and lungs, and has been associated with addictive processes, depression, amnesia, cancer, and pain. In addition, DMT also activates the TAAR1 receptor, known as the receptor associated with trace amines. Generally, the molecules that act as agonists to this receptor display anxiolytic, antipsychotic, and antiaddictive effects, explaining to some extent some of the therapeutic effects of DMT.

In the case of ayahuasca, we find ourselves before a more complex scenario. This is the result of the slow decoction of at least two plants, *Banisteriopsis caapi* (rich in the MAO inhibitors, beta-carbolines) and *Psychotria viridis* (rich in DMT), although literally dozens of other plants can be used to make a more or less similar drink. As natural products, we can deduce that there will be relevant concentrations of many different compounds in the resulting beverage. In addition to DMT, from the *P. viridis*, the beta-carbolines also have a rather complex mechanism of action, and that, of course, is not limited to MAO inhibition. These beta-carbolines, such as tetrahydroharmine or harmaline, also activate the receptor 5-HT1A and different types of the 5-HT2 subreceptor. In addition, they also activate the D2 receptor, the GABA receptors, the imidazoline I2 receptor, the adrenergic alpha-2 receptor, the benzodiazepine receptors, and the opioid receptors.

Ayahuasca contains mainly three beta-carbolines (tetrahydroharmine, harmine, and harmaline), and each has a somewhat characteristic binding profile. For example, harmine has higher affinity for the 5-HT2A receptor than the other beta-carbolines.

Beyond DMT and beta-carbolines, around two thousand more substances have been detected in ayahuasca, mainly phenolic compounds widely present in the plant kingdom. The implications that the presence of all these compounds may have on the therapeutic or psychoactive effects of ayahuasca is currently an unexplored field, since there are practically no studies that have elucidated the high complexity of this drink, beyond the associated effects of the presence of DMT and beta-carbolines.

ERGOLAMINE TARGETS

Ergolamines, like LSD, have a receptor binding profile very similar to those of simple tryptamines. As we have mentioned before, most of the compounds that can be considered "psychedelics" will bind mainly to serotonin receptors, especially 5-HT2A. Ergolamines are no exception.

TABLE 4. MAIN TARGETS OF LSD

LSD Targets	Ki
Serotonin receptors	
5-HT$_{1A}$	1.1
5-HT$_{1B}$	3.9
5-HT$_{1E}$	93
5-HT$_{2A}$	3.5
5-HT$_{2C}$	5.5
Histamine receptors	
H1	1,540
Adrenergic receptors	
alpha$_2$	37
beta$_1$	140
beta$_2$	740
Dopamine receptors	
D$_1$	180
D$_2$	120
D$_3$	27
D$_4$	56
D$_5$	340

LSD

LSD interacts with various serotonin receptors, including the following subreceptors: 5-HT1A, 5-HT1B, 5-HT1E, 5-HT2A, and 5-HT2C, among others. However, the binding profile of LSD with these receptors is somewhat peculiar. The molecule is not limited to binding and unbinding to the receptor, as usually happens, but once this binding occurs, the adjoining part of the receptor folds over the LSD molecule, forming a kind of "lid" that prevents the substance from detaching itself from the receptor. It is partly because of this latch that covers the LSD molecule that the psychoactive effects of this substance last for so many hours. About twelve hours after the substance has been ingested, part of the LSD detaches from the receptor, in those cases where the layer that covered it is modified. When this layer is not modified, the cell ends up absorbing the serotonin receptor together with the LSD, to degrade and reuse the materials.

Another difference, with respect to the simple tryptamines, is that LSD and other ergolamines have a higher affinity for dopamine receptors. Specifically, LSD has a high affinity for subreceptors D1, D2, D3, D4, and D5, although it acts as a partial agonist to D1 and D2 subreceptors. There is some evidence on the possible implication of dopamine receptors in the psychoactive effects of LSD. For example, the administration of moderate or high doses of chlorpromazine (a dopamine receptor antagonist; the first antipsychotic drug to be discovered and used in clinics) prevents some negative effects of LSD, such as nausea, dizziness, or anxiety, from manifesting without reducing its perceptual distortions. Additionally, LSD also binds to histamine and adrenergic receptors.

LSA

Few studies have been carried out with other ergolamines, such as LSA (ergine), although it is known that, despite also binding to serotonin and dopamine receptors, it does so with less affinity than LSD. It also appears to show affinity for a greater number of receptors, therefore being a more complex substance than LSD. For example, it binds to more adrenergic receptors (of adrenaline, an excitatory neurotransmitter), histamine (excitatory amine), muscarinic (receptors of the acetylcholine group), or serotonergic. This may be because LSA is a natural substance found in some plants, such as *Argyreia nervosa*, while LSD is a semisynthetic substance. Natural products, by definition, tend to interact with a large number of receptors.

PHENETHYLAMINE TARGETS

In this group we talk about two main substances: mescaline and MDMA. Although they are apparently very different substances (the first is basically present in different cacti used in religious/spiritual ceremonies, and the second is widely used recreationally, but also, less extensively, in psychotherapy), the truth is that they belong to the same pharmacological class of phenethylamines.

Mescaline

Mescaline is commonly described as a nonselective serotonin receptor agonist. This means that it is a molecule that is going to interact with many different types of serotonin receptors, primarily 5-HT1A, 5-HT2A, 5-HT2B, and 5-HT2C. It also presents a rather low affinity toward receptors alpha-2 and TAAR1. As we have seen with *Psilocybe* mushrooms, if mescaline is consumed by preparing cactus such as peyote (*Lophophora williamsii*) or San Pedro (*Echinopsis pachanoi*), many other substances will modulate the effect of mescaline, and significant differences in their psychoactive effects may be found.

MDMA

The binding profile of MDMA receptors differs quite a bit from that of mescaline. MDMA, or ecstasy, increases serotonin levels in the synaptic cleft, but somewhat indirectly and through different pathways. It has been observed that this substance is capable of inhibiting the serotonin transporter (SERT). Furthermore, when MDMA reaches the presynaptic neuron, it prevents the storage of serotonin in the synaptic vesicles, releasing large amounts of serotonin that, under normal conditions, would not have been released. In this way, by inhibiting serotonin transport proteins, which would regulate the presence of this neurotransmitter in the synaptic cleft, and with the massive release of serotonin from the presynaptic neuron, MDMA produces a serotonin cascade in the synaptic cleft. In addition to the serotonin transporter,

MDMA also inhibits other transporters and MAO, increasing dopamine or norepinephrine levels, although its effect is especially noticeable on serotonin.

In addition to this indirect effect on serotonin levels, MDMA also binds to various receptors, among which we find the serotonin 5-HT2B receptor, the muscarinic receptor M3, adrenergic receptors alpha-2A, alpha-2B, and alpha-2C, and, with lower affinity, dopamine D1 and D2 receptors.

TABLE 5. MAIN TARGETS OF MDMA

MDMA Targets	Ki
Serotonin receptors	
5-HT_{2B}	500
Histamine receptors	
HI	1,540
Adrenergic receptors	
alpha_{2A}	2,532
alpha_{2B}	1,785
alpha_{2C}	1,346
Imidazoline receptors	
I_1	219
Muscarinic receptors	
M_3	1,851
Dopamine receptors	
D_1	>10,000
D_2	>10,000

TARGETS OF NMDA RECEPTOR ANTAGONISTS, INCLUDING KETAMINE

Although the title of this section seems self-explanatory, substances that generally act as NMDA receptor antagonists also act on other receptors. Ketamine is perhaps the quintessential substance of this group. In addition to its obvious action on NMDA receptors, ketamine also blocks nicotinic receptors, which are highly involved in cognitive and addictive processes. Additionally, it is an agonist of the delta-, kappa-, and mu-opioid receptors, as well as the dopamine D2 receptor, and acts as an antagonist to 5-HT1 and 5-HT2 receptors. It also inhibits acetylcholinesterase, the enzyme responsible for oxidizing acetylcholine, a neurotransmitter associated with cognition and memory (by inhibiting acetylcholinesterase, acetylcholine levels are increased).

The case of ketamine and the name of this category reminds us, once again, that we will almost never be able to identify a substance by a single mechanism of action. The effects of ketamine were originally associated with its antagonism to NMDA receptors. However, its complex effects cannot be understood without paying attention to its full receptor binding profile.

TARGETS OF NEW TRYPTAMINES

"New tryptamines" began to appear in the middle of the last century and were the result of the discovery of the intense psychoactive effects of DMT and other molecules present in snuffs (powder that is inhaled intranasally) from South America. From the first experiences with these products, intense work has been done on the synthesis of derivatives of these molecules, such as DPT, DET, and DFT.

The truth is that an entire "psychonautic" subculture has emerged, keen on testing these substances and identifying chemical particularities supposedly associated with their different receptor binding profiles. The interested reader can go to the Erowid website or delve into the work carried out by Ann and Alexander Shulgin or David Nichols, the chemists who have synthesized the newest tryptamines and who have best described their pharmacological characteristics.

There is not much to say about targets of new tryptamines, since, unfortunately, and no matter how much it weighs on us, we will not be able to suggest a general receptor binding pattern of the substances belonging to this category. First, because there are many, many different substances, and, second, because each one of them has its unique characteristics, which, in addition, have been poorly studied, the information available in this regard is rather scarce. Still, we can present the receptor binding profile of some of these compounds for illustration.

Methylcybin (4-HO-MET), for example, was synthesized by Alexander Shulgin and binds with high affinity to dopamine D1 and D3 receptors, as well as the dopamine transporter, DAT, increasing dopamine levels in the synaptic cleft. This high affinity for dopamine receptors is somewhat strange, since both its structure and its effects would suggest that it is primarily a serotonin receptor agonist. Albeit with lower affinity, it also binds to the adrenergic receptor alpha-1, to receptor TAAR1, to histamine receptor H1, or serotonin receptors 5-HT1A, 5-HT2A, and 5-HT2C.

DALT, or N,N-diallyltryptamine, is another new tryptamine that, in this case, binds mainly to serotonin receptors, although it also binds to some quite unusual subreceptors in the case of psychedelic tryptamines, such as 5-HT1B, 5-HT5A, and 5-HT6. Therefore the effects can be quite different with respect to those of simple tryptamines. It also binds to the 5-HT2A receptor, but with lower affinity. In addition to these serotonin receptors, it inhibits SERT and DAT. As for adrenergic receptors, it binds to the receptor alpha-1D with high affinity and others with less affinity. It binds with high affinity to dopamine D1, D2, D4, and D5 receptors, as well as mu- and delta-opioid receptors (also to kappa-opioid receptors but with lower affinity). Lastly, regarding histamine H1 and H2 receptors, it does the same but with great affinity.

As can be clearly seen, the group of substances that can be considered new tryptamines contains molecules that present quite unusual receptor binding profiles and that represent authentic exceptions in the field of psychedelic drugs. These substances are, on the one hand, an opportunity to explore new therapeutic approaches that should be taken advantage of and thoroughly explored, and, on the other, a possible source of accidents and unwanted effects, mainly due to the lack of information on toxicity or long-term effects. In any case, we must keep in mind that in this category we are going to find very heterogeneous binding profiles and that we will rarely be able to include these molecules under the same pattern.

TARGETS OF ATYPICAL PSYCHEDELICS

Surely the fact that some psychedelics have been classified as "atypical" drugs responds to different misconceptions. For example, it is possible to question, from the outset, the inclusion within the same "psychedelic" category of different drugs that are absolutely and completely different, but that induce dramatic changes in the state of consciousness of those who consume them. The type of alterations in the state of consciousness that could be considered as characteristic of psychedelic drugs have not yet been defined. Nor is there a criterion that establishes where these would end and other types of alterations of consciousness, that are not strictly psychedelic, would begin, since there is a wide range of substances, from caffeine to propofol, that alter our state of consciousness in one way or another. Therefore, inside the mixed bag of psychedelic drugs, we may find some strange items that surely should not be there. Or maybe this category should not even exist, but that's another question entirely.

Ibogaine/Noribogaine

We can consider ibogaine/noribogaine as the quintessential atypical psychedelic, because it has several mechanisms of action clearly absent in other psychedelic drugs. Instead of just mentioning ibogaine, which is the naturally occurring alkaloid found in the root of *T. iboga* and other plants, we will comment on its binding profile and that of noribogaine, its major metabolite when metabolized in the human body. Noribogaine plays a crucial role both in explaining the general effects of ibogaine and its possible therapeutic effects, so we would fall short if we focused only on the main molecule.

Both ibogaine and noribogaine bind to the opioid receptors, and they do so in a very particular way. Both act as mu-receptor antagonists, but ibogaine exerts a much more potent antagonistic action at this receptor. In contrast, while both are kappa-receptor agonists, it is noribogaine that activates this receptor more strongly. Given that ibogaine remains in blood circulation for only a few hours, after which noribogaine appears to stay up to several days, we can appreciate the peculiar dynamics in the activation of opioid receptors. While shortly after consuming ibogaine we will have a strong mu-receptor antagonism and a mild kappa-receptor agonism, as the hours progress, this state will be reversed, turning into a powerful kappa-receptor agonism and an attenuated mu-receptor antagonism.

There are three main opioid receptors: mu, delta, and kappa. Most opioids with euphoric and addictive effects, such as heroin, are mu-receptor agonists. However, kappa-receptor agonists tend to cause aversive effects and, in fact, have antiaddictive effects.

Once ingested, ibogaine inhibits dopamine and serotonin transporters, increasing the levels of these neurotransmitters in the synaptic cleft, although without presenting relevant affinities for direct binding to their receptors. It should be noted that noribogaine inhibits SERT with a potency 10 times higher than ibogaine, so serotonin levels increase as ibogaine is metabolized. Both substances, ibogaine and its metabolite, also act as NMDA receptor antagonists (like ketamine), and at the nicotinic subreceptor alpha-3 beta-4, widely associated with addictive behaviors. In fact, antagonist medicines for this subreceptor are highly promising for the treatment of substance use disorders.

We should also highlight ibogaine's capacity to inhibit ATP-dependent membrane transporters (also known as ABCs). Specifically, ibogaine has been shown to inhibit P-glycoprotein (P-gp) and the breast cancer resistance protein (BCRP). These proteins are responsible for the expulsion of exogenous molecules from cells. They are a kind of barrier

TABLE 6. MAIN TARGETS OF IBOGAINE
AND NORIBOGAINE

Targets of ibogaine	Ki	Targets of noribogaine	Ki
SERT	0.2	SERT	5.26
DAT	1.98	DAT	2.05
Sigma receptors			
Sigma$_2$	0.2	Sigma$_2$	5.26
Opioid receptors			
Mu	3.76	Mu	0.16
Kappa	3.77	Kappa	0.96
Glutamate receptors			
NMDA	5.2	NMDA	31
Cholinergic receptors			
Alpha3-beta4	1.05	Alpha3-beta4	-

that prevents potentially dangerous substances from gaining access to the interior of the cells, which is why both P-gp and BCRP are highly associated with the phenomenon of tolerance or resistance to multiple drugs, even when the resistance is not desirable, such as when receiving drug therapy for infectious diseases, cancer, or other illnesses. P-gp and BCRP are present in multiple tissues, but especially in those that are critical for the separation of vital structures and organs that the body constantly tries to protect against toxins, such as the blood-brain barrier, the epithelial cells of the intestine, or the intrahepatic bile ducts. When we develop tolerance to some substance or drug, such as opioids or cannabis, the concentrations of this type of transport proteins increase, with the aim of expelling the molecules of these substances.

This is one of the reasons why higher doses are needed to induce the same effect: there are more and more carrier proteins capable of expelling these substances. Thus, the inhibitory action of ibogaine on these proteins may be partially related to the reduction in drug tolerance observed in users, who consistently report that, after taking ibogaine, they need to take much fewer doses of other drugs to feel the same effects. But this is not limited to drugs like cocaine or heroin; it also happens with caffeine and nicotine.

We were able to repeatedly observe this phenomenon in an ibogaine clinical study carried out in the city of Reus, Spain. Several participants unintentionally drastically reduced their consumption of tobacco or coffee during the study, although the intended outcome was to discontinue their methadone use.

For those interested in delving deeper in the mechanisms of action of ibogaine, we have published a narrative review on that regard.[6] Also, with Judit Biosca and Teresa Colomina we have published the first transcriptomic study on ibogaine in order to explore unknown genetic alterations produced by this substance.[7]

Salvinorin-A

Salvinorin-A is quite a mystery, not only within the group of psychedelic compounds but in pharmacology in general. First, because it is, without a doubt, among the most powerful psychedelic substances of plant origin, not being an alkaloid, but a terpene. Generally, plant compounds with psychoactive properties are alkaloids (cocaine, morphine, and mescaline, among others). Only in *C. sativa* (cannabinoids are not alkaloids either), *S. divinorum*, and a few other uncharacteristic plants do we find psychoactive compounds that are not alkaloids.

6. Ona G, Reverte I, Rossi GN, et al. 2023. Main targets of ibogaine and noribogaine associated with its putative anti-addictive effects: a mechanistic overview. Journal of Psychopharmacology 37(12):1190–1200.

7. Biosca-Brull J, Ona G, Alarcón-Franco L, Colomina MT. 2024. A transcriptomic analysis in mice following a single dose of ibogaine identifies new potential therapeutic targets. Translational Psychiatry 14(41).

In addition to this unusual characteristic, it is also extremely unusual for a molecule of natural origin to have such a selective action in our organism, since salvinorin-A binds primarily and with high affinity to the kappa-opioid receptor, acting as a potent agonist. It seems exclusively designed for this receptor, since it does not even affect other opioid receptors, as is often the case with substances that bind to these receptors. Opioid receptors tend to form complexes, so the vast majority of substances that bind to them affect more than one type of receptor. Mu-receptor agonists, for example, also have a certain action on delta or kappa receptors, making it very difficult to find ligands that bind only to a specific receptor. An exception is the case of salvinorin-A, which only affects kappa receptors. This can be explained because, in fact, its molecular structure is completely different from that of the rest of the opiate ligands. In figure 20 we can observe the unusual selectivity of salvinorin-A compared to LSD.

There is yet another peculiarity. Opioid receptor agonists tend to downregulate these receptors. This means that when these receptors are activated as a result of the binding to opiate molecules, some of them cease to be functional. It is believed that because this population of receptors can detect when there is a large number of molecules with an affinity to them, many are deactivated to avoid possible saturation or dysfunction of the system. So after being exposed to morphine or codeine, for example, the body will regulate itself so that only a few of the opioid receptors "receive" more opiate molecules (something that is also related, by the way, to tolerance, since with fewer and fewer receptors available, the same effect is not achieved as the first time these substances were consumed). Well, it turns out that salvinorin-A, despite being a potent agonist, does not significantly downregulate kappa-opioid receptors, suggesting that it does not induce tolerance.

Beyond these peculiar properties, to say the least, and its affinity for the kappa-opioid receptor, it has also been observed that salvinorin-A has some agonist activity on the dopamine D2 receptor, although quite weak. Moreover, it also appears to activate the dopamine transporter (thus reducing dopamine concentrations in the synaptic cleft) and inhibit SERT.

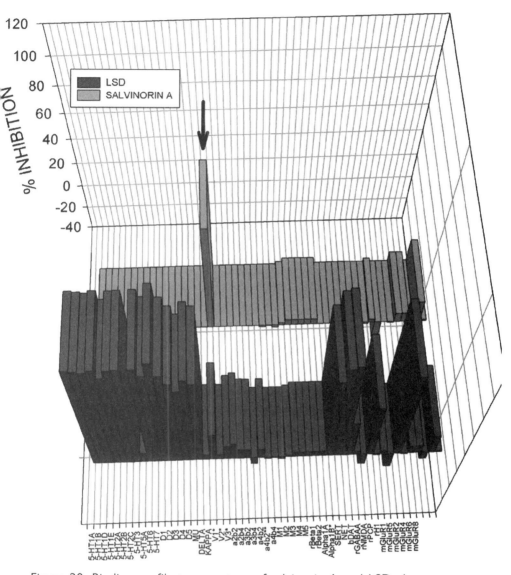

Figure 20. Binding profile to receptors of salvinorin-A and LSD. As you can see, while LSD shows affinity for a large number of receptors, salvinorin-A is highly selective and only shows a high affinity for the kappa-opioid receptor. Original image from the article: Roth BL, Baner K, Westkaemper R, Siebert D, Rice KC, Steinberg S, Ernsberger P, Rothman RB. 2002. Salvinorin A: a potent, naturally occurring, non-nitrogenous kappa-opioid selective agonist. Proceedings of the National Academy of Sciences of the United States of America 99(18):11934–11939. Reproduced with authors' permission.

Datura stramonium

It is convenient to talk about this plant as a whole, since its active principles have not been extracted and commercialized in its pure form, as has been done in the case of *T. iboga* and *S. divinorum*, probably because of its unpleasant effects and its high toxicity. There are also no notable differences in their mechanisms of action, so we are actually talking about quite similar molecules.

The main psychoactive compounds of *D. stramonium* are scopolamine, hyoscyamine, and atropine, which are found in large quantities in the seeds of the plant. These are part of the group of tropane alkaloids, so named because they contain a tropane ring in their molecular structure. Although scopolamine and atropine are usually the most abundant compounds, hyoscyamine and about sixty other tropane alkaloids are also present in the plant and may also play a role in the final effects.

Scopolamine, hyoscyamine, and atropine are potent muscarinic receptor antagonists in general. They are part of the cholinergic neurotransmission system and therefore these alkaloids are generally defined as anticholinergics, because they block the neurotransmission of acetylcholine. Because muscarinic receptors are widely associated with cognitive processes, antagonists of these receptors have been associated with detrimental effects on cognition. They also act, especially scopolamine, as 5-HT3 receptor antagonists, which are used to relieve nausea, vomiting, and dizziness, possibly explaining the therapeutic applications of scopolamine. This is the alkaloid that binds most strongly to muscarinic receptors, while hyoscyamine is the alkaloid with the weakest effect on them.

REFERENCES FOR FURTHER STUDY

Cameron LP, Olson DE. 2018. Dark classics in chemical neuroscience: N,N-dimethyltryptamine (DMT). ACS Chemical Neuroscience 9(10):2344–2357.

Cassels BK, Sáez-Briones P. 2018. Dark classics in chemical neuroscience: mescaline. ACS Chemical Neuroscience 9(10):2448–2458.

Dunlap LE, Andrews AM, Olson DE. 2018. Dark classics in chemical neuroscience: 3,4-methylenedioxymethamphetamine. ACS Chemical Neuroscience 9(10):2408–2427.

Hernández-Alvarado RB, Madariaga-Mazón A, Ortega A, Martínez-Mayorga K. 2020. Dark classics in chemical neuroscience: salvinorin A. ACS Chemical Neuroscience Dec 2;11(23):3979–3992.

Holze F, Singh N, Liechti ME, D'Souza DC. 2024. Serotonergic Psychedelics—a comparative review comparing the efficacy, safety, pharmacokinetics and binding profile of serotonergic psychedelics. Biological Psychiatry: Cognitive Neuroscience and Neuroimaging Jan 30:S2451-9022(24)00020-X.

Katchborian-Neto A, Santos WT, Nicacio KJ, Correa JOA, Murgu M, Paula ACC. 2020. Neuroprotective potential of ayahuasca and untargeted metabolomics analyses: applicability to Parkinson's disease. Journal of Ethnopharmacology 255:112743.

Lakstygal AM, Kolesnikova TO, Khatsko SL, Zabegalov KN, Volgin AD, Demin KA, Shevyrin VA, Wappler-Guzzetta EA, Kalueff AV. 2019. Dark classics in chemical neuroscience: atropine, scopolamine, and other anticholinergic deliriant hallucinogens. ACS Chemical Neuroscience 10(5):2144–2159.

Maehle AH. 2009. A binding question: the evolution of the receptor concept. Endeavour 33(4):135–140.

Roth BL. 2006. The serotonin receptors: from molecular pharmacology to human therapeutics. Totowa (NJ): Humana Press.

Wacker D, Wang S, McCorvy JD, Betz RM, Venkatakrishnan AJ, Levit A, Lansu K, Schools ZL, Che T, Nichols DE, Shoichet BK, Dror RO, Roth BL. 2017. Crystal structure of an LSD-bound human serotonin receptor. Cell 168(3):377–389.e12.

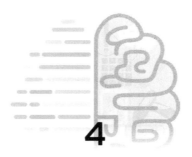

4

Characteristic Aspects of Psychedelics Pharmacology

The biggest myth about psychedelics is precisely the belief that by taking them you will have a psychedelic experience, when what really happens is that you have a greater human experience, a greater experience of yourself.

RICK DOBLIN

This chapter constitutes one of the central (and, therefore, also the densest) parts of this book, where the most characteristic aspects of the pharmacology of different psychedelic drugs will be properly explained. In pharmacology, the concepts of pharmacokinetics and pharmacodynamics are absolutely essential. They are the cornerstone of any pharmacological description. It is the best way that has been found to quickly map how any drug acts in our body. Pharmacokinetics, for example, is considered the identifying mark, the fingerprint, of any molecule. When the patents on new drugs expire (after ten to fifteen years from their authorization) and the active ingredients of the drugs are marketed under other brands, known as "generic" drugs, pharmacokinetic studies are then undertaken to test if the generic is the same drug as the drug that had been used under the patent. If both molecules are absorbed, distributed, and processed in the body in the same way, then it can be said that the generic and the "brand" drug are absolutely the same.

This chapter will be divided into two sections. Each will offer a detailed explanation of the concepts of pharmacokinetics and pharmacodynamics, respectively, using psychedelic drugs as examples. The idea is for the reader to learn the fundamentals of pharmacology in an entertaining way and, incidentally, learn how these fundamentals relate to psychedelics. Proceeding in the reverse order would have required working on the basis of repetitive and redundant lists, creating a text that was more of a reference, not very suitable for continuous reading. Thus, the reader will also be able to apply the general knowledge of pharmacology they may acquire here, not only to psychedelic drugs but also to medicines in general, resulting in greater empowerment and more informed decisions when using them. Perhaps the chosen formula is not perfect, but it is the best that the chaotic functioning of the author's neurons was able to devise.

Pharmacokinetics

The definition of the concept of pharmacokinetics was already explained in the first chapter of the book in a general way, but we can reintroduce it by saying that it includes all the processes to which exogenous molecules are exposed when they enter the body. These processes, in fact, serve the function of protecting the organism from foreign substances. Our body tries by all means to restrict the effect of any foreign substance. It is because of this that it processes, breaks, and excretes all the molecules that it does not recognize as its own, in addition to limiting their access to certain areas of the body using numerous barriers (the intestinal epithelium, the cell membrane, the skin, the blood-brain barrier, and others).

All the steps through which exogenous molecules pass have been divided into five main stages (release, absorption, distribution, metabolism, and excretion), giving rise to the acronym RADME, although ADME is also often spoken of, which does not consider the release.

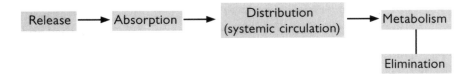

Figure 21. Phases of RADME (release, absorption, distribution, metabolism, and elimination). Each of these stages is explained in detail in later sections.

The study of these stages allows not only a better understanding of the tortuous life of these poor molecules, but also the rational design of drugs with the intention of reducing their adverse effects and increasing their efficacy. For example, the cardiotoxic potential of ibogaine is well known. It has been suggested, although currently there is no evidence for this, that the administration of plant extracts containing ibogaine instead of the isolated pure molecule can reduce its cardiotoxicity, as has been observed in other natural products with similar effects on cardiac function. The hypothesis that an extract may be safer than an isolated molecule stems precisely from the pharmacokinetic knowledge of this class of products, since the interaction of the product's compounds may, on occasion, allow slower absorption, mitigate some side effects, or improve the metabolism of the active principle causing the effects on the heart.

Other factors that can influence the pharmacokinetics of a product or substance are its molecular size and structure, its solubility, or its plasma protein binding profile. In terms of size, the smaller the molecule, the more it will be absorbed and distributed in the body, suffering less from the effects of its various barriers. Most psychedelics consist of small molecules, so, a priori, we can think that most of them are absorbed with some ease. Regarding solubility, it is also true that molecules that are very lipid soluble (easily soluble in fat), also called non-polar, will more easily cross these barriers, while polar substances, with a profile that is more soluble in water (water soluble), will have a harder time crossing these barriers and therefore will be absorbed with greater difficulty. Again, most psychedelics are nonpolar. In the case of psilocybin, for example, it is quite water soluble, so it is not easily absorbed and practically does not reach the CNS. However, psilocybin is metabolized to form psilocin, which is much more fat soluble and ends up being the main cause of the psychoactive effects of psilocybin mushrooms.

Another key factor in pharmacokinetics is the plasma protein binding of the molecule in question. This refers to the fact that, once the exogenous substance is absorbed and therefore enters the bloodstream, being distributed throughout the body, a part of these exogenous molecules will bind to proteins in our blood, mainly albumin, because it is the most abundant circulating protein in our blood. This binding to proteins will limit the bioavailability of the substance, that is, the fraction that ends up being pharmacologically active, since only "free" molecules, not bound to proteins, will end up binding to their site of action (receptors or other targets). This is a truly paradoxical situation. Exogenous molecules need to access the bloodstream to distribute themselves and deploy their effects, but the price they pay to enter the bloodstream is that a fraction of them have to remain attached to the proteins present in the bloodstream, thereby they are unable to reach their destination. Most psychedelics bind effectively to plasma proteins, although without affecting their action in a relevant way.

INITIAL PHASES OF THE PROCESSING OF PSYCHEDELICS

Like with any other drug, the initial phases of our body's processing of psychedelic drugs play an essential role in the subsequent effects these substances may have. In later sections we will delve deep into such effects. Next, we will introduce these initial phases, providing examples of different psychedelic drugs and their particularities.

Release

In the case of psychedelic drugs, the release phase of the substance is rarely going to be relevant. In the case of medicines, for example, the release consists of the dissolution of the capsule or tablet that has been ingested, so that the tissues can absorb its content. As for LSD, for example, this is produced instantaneously by sucking on blotter paper, exposing the buccal mucosa to LSD, and allowing direct access to the bloodstream without passing through the stomach or other tissues, although a fraction of it will still end up passing through the stomach. In the case of ayahuasca or liquid psychedelics, no release is necessary, since the liquid format of the substance already allows its absorption. Psychedelics that are commonly presented in tablet form, such as MDMA in some cases, would follow the general release model consistent with most drugs. In this case, a parameter that should be calculated to describe the efficacy of its release would be the time it takes for the tablet to dissolve in humid and acidic environments such as the stomach and how possible adulterants or impurities present in the tablet affect this process.

Absorption

Once the psychedelic in question has entered our body and has been released, the absorption phase begins. Absorption and bioavailability are two concepts that go hand in hand. The bioavailability is the fraction of the drug or substance that ends up reaching the site of action and, generally, this will depend on the efficiency of the absorption process.

Substances that are administered orally, for example, are going to be absorbed by the gastrointestinal tract and, depending on the pH conditions, physicochemical properties (solubility), or metabolism, its absorption can be more or less efficient. For example, some substances are metabolized by the liver and are excreted in the bile without entering the systemic circulation. In this case we would speak of a null absorption. The metabolism of the liver and intestine are the main areas of "processing" of drugs or substances, and their passage through them is called first-pass metabolism. In the presence of any type of liver failure, various pharmacokinetic processes are affected. For example, in advanced stages of liver disease, a significant portion of the blood in the portal vein bypasses the liver and flows directly into the systemic circulation. This causes all drugs that have a significant first-pass metabolism (in the case of psychedelics, we can mention ayahuasca, ibogaine, or MDMA) to pass directly into the bloodstream, substantially increasing their concentrations and therefore generating a higher risk of intoxication. On the other hand, intravenous administration allows, in most cases, for all of the administered substance to reach the site of action precisely because first-pass metabolism is avoided.

In some diseases or special conditions, the absorption can also be considerably altered. This is the case with Crohn's disease, people who have undergone gastric resections, or those with diarrhea. In these cases, people do not absorb many drugs or substances very well, and it may be one of the reasons why notable psychoactive effects are not felt with moderate or high doses.

Most psychedelic drugs are administered orally. For example, once psilocybin is ingested and passes through the gastrointestinal tract, it is metabolized in the liver producing psilocin, a substance that passes into the systemic circulation and produces psychoactive effects. It is certainly noteworthy that the liver enzymes responsible for its metabolism are still not exactly known, and surprisingly, not many studies have been published on the human metabolism of psilocybin. Psilocin, in turn, after being distributed throughout the body, including the brain, re-enters the liver and the small intestine, where it is again metabolized, and finally excreted through the kidneys. It should be noted that this process has been studied using synthetic psilocybin, so consuming psilocybin mushrooms surely works somewhat differently, with many other substances accompanying psilocybin, including MAO inhibitors, which suggests greater bioavailability of psilocybin/psilocin when mushrooms are ingested, although future studies will need to elucidate this question.

DMT can be consumed in various ways. The smoke resulting

from the vaporization of DMT extracted from plants that contain it is generally inhaled and, of course, it is also consumed orally through ayahuasca. Some studies were carried out as early as the seventies of the last century, administering pure DMT to healthy volunteers through intramuscular or intravenous injections, at doses between 0.05 and 0.4 mg per kilo of weight. Intramuscular administration produced somewhat delayed effects (the peak of psychoactive effects was reached about ten minutes after injection), while intravenous injection produced psychoactive effects almost instantaneously. It was observed, as is well known today, that DMT is rapidly metabolized, and in a matter of sixty to ninety minutes it almost completely disappears from blood plasma, although the concentrations are already very low thirty minutes after administration. Something similar happens when the smoke resulting from the vaporization of DMT is inhaled, since gastrointestinal metabolism is avoided through the lungs and access to systemic circulation is practically instantaneous, as the surface of the lung is very extensive and the smoke covers much of the organ once inhaled through the lungs, reaching all mucous membranes and the pulmonary epithelium. The same is true of other substances that are also vaporized and inhaled through the lungs, such as 5-MeO-DMT (although this can also be inhaled through the nose), salvinorin-A, or changa (a mixture of naturally extracted DMT and various plants).

The absorption pattern of DMT is drastically modified when it is ingested orally through ayahuasca. The beta-carbolines present in ayahuasca inhibit the first-pass metabolism that would completely eliminate the absorption of DMT if it were administered orally, so that it can be absorbed and reach significant concentrations in blood plasma thirty to forty minutes after ingestion, disappearing almost completely after six to eight hours.

LSD is also usually administered orally, although the sublingual route is often recommended. In the case of following such recommendations, the concentrations of LSD in blood plasma would begin to appear after a few minutes of placing the blotter paper under the tongue.

MDMA can be presented in powder or tablet form, as different

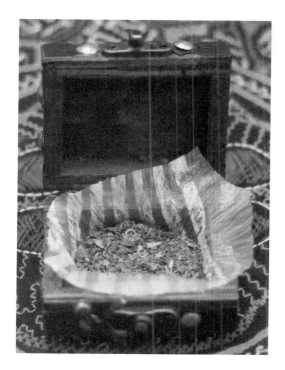

Figure 22. Photograph of "changa," a product where synthetic DMT is mixed with different plants, such as the blue lotus (*Nymphaea caerulea*) or *Peganum harmala*. Photograph courtesy of Sebastián Troncoso.

salts increase the solubility and stability of the molecule, the most common being the hydrochloride salt. This format allows the substance to be ingested orally, either in the form of tablets or through "bombs" (small amounts of powder wrapped in cigarette paper) or by directly inhaling the powder. As for nasal aspiration, it could be considered as effective as the pulmonary route, as it quickly facilitates access to the mucous membranes. However, it should be noted that it is a much less effective route, since metabolizing enzymes are also present in the nasal mucosa, so not all of the substance will be absorbed "cleanly." It is also true that the surface is much smaller than the lungs, so it fills up quickly and prevents the entire amount aspirated from being absorbed. In addition, the mucus that is present may also plug the entrance to the mucosa (not to mention the feeling is not very pleasant). When MDMA is ingested orally, it is absorbed mainly in the intestine and takes about two hours to reach the maximum concentration in the blood.

Ketamine can also be administered through different routes, although the most common in recreational contexts is to inhale it. In clinical, therapeutic, and personal growth settings, it is usually injected intramuscularly or, to a lesser extent, intravenously, although techniques have also been developed for its intranasal application. Intramuscular injections are highly effective, with a bioavailability greater than 90 percent, reaching peak plasma concentration after five minutes. Intravenous injection is, of course, also highly effective. When ingested orally, bioavailability is drastically reduced due to first-pass metabolism, reaching around 20 percent. When the intranasal route is used, bioavailability is 50 percent. Nevertheless, it has been the preferred method for clinical use in the case of esketamine (the "S" enantiomer of ketamine; [S]-ketamine) for addressing treatment-resistant depression, as it is a less invasive route.

Mescaline is usually taken orally with beverages made from peyote or San Pedro. Therefore, it is absorbed through the gastrointestinal tract. Interestingly, a large amount of mescaline is rapidly stored in the liver and kidney, being released slowly, which delays the onset of effects and the elimination of the substance. Actually, in some animal studies, higher proportions of mescaline have been observed in the liver and kidney than in the brain. This may be due, in part, to the fact that mescaline is poorly lipid soluble, which makes it difficult for it to cross some of the aforementioned barriers, such as the blood-brain barrier. Therefore, much higher doses than those of other psychedelics are also necessary to induce psychoactive effects.

In the case of ibogaine, it is consumed in different formats, although always orally. We can find extracts from *T. iboga*, purified extracts with high content of ibogaine, as well as synthetic ibogaine. Both this substance and its main metabolite, noribogaine, are highly fat soluble and are able to cross barriers, both gaining easy access to the brain, unlike psilocybin and psilocin. An important portion of ibogaine goes to bind to plasma proteins, so quite high doses are also needed to induce intense psychoactive effects. Ibogaine undergoes extensive first-pass metabolism, during which noribogaine is produced. It is important to note

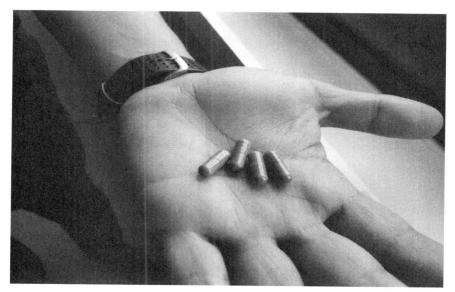

Figure 23. Ibogaine capsules to be administered orally, in the context of a clinical trial developed at the Hospital Universitari Sant Joan de Reus in Spain, for the treatment of methadone dependence.
Photograph taken and provided by the author.

that important differences in absorption between genders have been found. Plasma concentrations of ibogaine can be up to 3 times higher in women than in men, showing 43 percent bioavailability in men and 71 percent in women.

Atropine and the rest of the tropane alkaloids are rapidly absorbed regardless of the route of administration, only varying the time of appearance of the effects. In addition, scopolamine, being more powerful, can be applied in patches on the skin or transdermal.

Distribution

This phase of pharmacokinetics summarizes the passage of the drug or substance throughout our body, since once absorption has been successfully carried out, the molecules have entered systemic circulation and are freely distributed to organs and tissues. Some factors must be taken into account, which will affect this distribution and therefore can alter the presence of the substance in some parts of our body.

In the first place, as is evident, the distribution basically depends on the bloodstream, since this is in fact its means of transport. If circulation is disturbed in any way, distribution will be too. For example, if the heart rate is very high, distribution will be greater, the substance will reach the sites of action sooner, and its effects will be established more quickly. In this sense, another factor that will influence distribution is the regional blood flow, the volume of blood that reaches each organ or tissue, the most irrigated being the ones most exposed to the substance. Some examples can be seen in Table 7, but we could say that the most irrigated organs are the liver, the kidney, and the brain.

TABLE 7. DISTRIBUTION OF BLOOD FLOW

	Kidneys	Heart	Liver	Brain	Skeletal muscles	Fat
Blood Flow (mL/min)	1,100	250	1,700	800	900	250
Mass (kg)	0.3	0.3	2.6	1.3	3.4	10
% Cardiac Output	20	4.5	31	14.5	16.4	4.5

The inherent characteristics of each molecule will also affect its distribution, as has been previously mentioned. Thus, highly lipophilic molecules will distribute into the CNS with ease, whereas those that are not so lipophilic will perhaps have their distribution restricted to the peripheral nervous system (PNS). Albumin levels in each person will also be relevant[1] in cases where a significant fraction of the drug or substance binds to plasma proteins. In diseases that occur with inflammatory processes or in people with nutritional deficiencies, albumin levels will be low, and therefore there will be more "free" molecules, increasing the effects of the substance.

---

1. Albumin is the most abundant protein in the blood. It is produced in the liver and is involved in multiple functions.

It is also noteworthy that aging considerably alters distribution. Over the years, our body loses muscle tissue, increases the total percentage of fat, and decreases body water. This causes highly lipophilic substances to increase their distribution and prolong their half-life, while hydrophilic substances will have a more limited distribution. Beyond the field of psychedelics, this should be taken into account in daily clinical practice and lower doses should be prescribed of fat-soluble drugs (which are, moreover, the vast majority). However, the dosage is rarely adapted to elderly patients, exposing them to intoxications that lead to symptoms of dementia or other serious side effects.

There are not many differences with respect to the pattern of distribution between the different psychedelic substances. It would only be necessary to take into account the special cases of psilocybin, which, as the reader may know by now, has a rather limited distribution, and it will be psilocin, its metabolite, that will be more widely distributed by the CNS, or mescaline, which also has a limited distribution and is quite restricted to the liver and kidney, and therefore high doses are needed to achieve psychoactive effects. The highly lipophilic profile of ibogaine and noribogaine is also remarkable, perhaps one of the most remarkable. This means that they are rapidly distributed throughout the CNS and that their concentrations are disproportionately higher in regions of this system, mainly the brain. For example, concentrations of ibogaine have been found to be up to 100 times higher in fat tissue than can be found in plasma, and in the brain up to 30 times higher than in plasma.

METABOLISM

The human body relies on metabolism for two main tasks: to properly process and absorb nutrients from our diet, and to remove foreign substances (also called xenobiotics) that are toxic or potentially toxic to our body, so that they do not accumulate and end up causing damage to a tissue or organ. In the past, both humans and other animals were constantly exposed to potentially lethal toxins, mainly of plant origin. In order to eliminate these substances effectively and thus avoid repeated fatalities that would have endangered a species, human and animal metabolism gradually specialized to combat a wide range of exogenous substances. Therefore, the function of metabolism is to protect us, and its job is to expel any xenobiotic that accesses our body.

Plants are specialists in producing chemicals that can affect the behavior of animals, including humans. As we explained in chapter 1, the secondary metabolites that are produced in plants have the sole objective of altering the behavior of their predators and, if possible, even killing them. We will consider this scenario in a little more detail to understand the functions of certain secondary metabolites and their interaction with animal metabolism.

Let's place ourselves on our planet, forty or fifty million years ago. The plant kingdom is already quite developed and coexists with different animals of different species that can move, climb, grab, and break whatever they want, including the poor plants, which cannot move and are, apparently, at a clear disadvantage. We say apparently because in reality, although they seem harmless, they have spent millions of years perfecting their chemical factories and are more than prepared to fight any animal that comes near them. On the other hand, these animals, as we've said, have also been subjected to a Darwinian selection for millions of years, which means that only those that are capable of metabolizing toxic plant substances survive and reproduce, ensuring and perpetuating these traits.

We therefore have in our scenario a growing population of animals resistant to the defense systems of plants. However, these plants, in turn, are also subject to the same laws of Darwin, so some of these plants start producing chemicals capable of inhibiting the metabolism of many animals and small organisms, so that, if their metabolism is inhibited, the toxic substances they produce will continue to affect and kill animals, just as it occurred before they learned to defend themselves. There is evolutionary pressure for the plants that produce these metabolism-inhibiting chemicals to survive, so their numbers begin to increase as well.

That is how today, just as we did in that scenario fifty million years ago, we have a profusion of plants that synthesize chemicals solely intended to inhibit metabolic systems, that is, defense systems. These chemicals are, for example, 5'-methoxyhydnocarpine, which is synthesized in many plants and inhibits chemical extrusion pumps present in soil pathogens; beta-carbolines also present in many other plants, such as *B. caapi*, which inhibit an essential enzyme in the metabolism of nutrients and xenobiotics, such as MAO; and ibogaine, inhibitor of P-gp and other membrane transport proteins, so crucial in the defense against xenobiotics and in the preservation of the integrity of CNS structures.

> It is thanks to the evolutionary pressure exerted on plants, to defend themselves from animals that wanted to eat them, that today we can temporarily inhibit our metabolism to effectively intoxicate ourselves with ayahuasca.

In general, xenobiotics are fat-soluble substances that, in the absence of metabolic processes, would accumulate in our body until some of our basic functions collapsed, causing death. Substances that are fat soluble do not pass easily into the aqueous environment that constitutes urine, so metabolism, in general terms, acts by modifying the structure of these substances to make them more water soluble and thus more easily eliminated through urine or bile. This is what happens in general terms, because sometimes the opposite can occur: metabolism may produce even more toxic or pharmacologically active substances, as is the case with psilocybin (which gives rise to psilocin, biologically active) or MDMA. In the latter case, if MDMA or MDA is administered directly to the brain, we would only observe a greater release of amines, such as serotonin or dopamine, but no neurotoxic effects, as occurs when MDMA is ingested orally and is metabolized in the liver. This suggests that the neurotoxicity associated with MDMA and other similar substances is more related to metabolic by-products generated in the liver and not to toxic actions directly produced by these substances. In fact, some of these metabolites have been isolated and administered in animal models, observing neurotoxic effects similar to those produced when MDMA is consumed orally (for example, long-term cognitive deficits and greater impulsivity).

Metabolism and Aging

At this point, aware as we now are of the function and complexity of metabolism, we must make a brief note about the changes it undergoes throughout life. Unfortunately, as years go by, metabolism does not perform its functions as effectively and it becomes progressively more incapable of processing and eliminating toxins or xenobiotics from the body. This has repercussions. For example, there is a greater probability of suffering adverse reactions derived from pharmacological intoxications, either relatively acute (for example, dizziness, falls, ulcers, and bleeding) or chronic, causing damage to the function of organs such as the liver or kidneys. A worse metabolism not only results in a notable increase in the harmful effects of the substance but also in a remarkable prolongation of the half-life. In fact, perhaps one of the most important reasons for mortality is precisely the progressive inefficiency of the body to metabolize drugs or toxic by-products in the body.

This suggests, again, that the doses (of any product) should be adjusted for those sixty-five or seventy years of age or older. For example, the most effective and safest dose of paracetamol for an adult is between 500 and 650 mg. An elderly person should use between 300 and 400 mg. Higher doses, which are unfortunately commonly used, will only result in more liver damage and not in greater efficacy, since efficacy has a "ceiling," but toxicity does not. In the case of psychoactive substances, the administered doses should also be lower than those usually used in adults. For example, in MDMA therapy, between 75 and 125 mg are commonly used. This suggests that, in the case of the elderly population, doses higher than 60 mg should not be administered. In this sense, there are not enough studies that can corroborate these recommendations. However, based on the knowledge we have of the functioning and deterioration of metabolic functions as we age, we should be cautious and not expose ourselves to potential toxic effects that are, in actuality, unnecessary.

I am very sorry to tell my readers over thirty years of age that it is from this age on that all the metabolic functions of the body begin to decline. As can be seen in figure 24, not only basal metabolism, but also the percentage of body water or kidney functions begin to decline. There is no special reason that leads to this progressive decline from the age of thirty; however, in an evolutionary context, it can be understood that the objective of our body and our genetics has not been to live a greater number of years, but rather of adapting to a hostile and constantly changing environment. To achieve such adaptation, human evolution has struck a delicate balance between the internal stability and homeostasis[2] necessary to carry out physiological functions that are essential for life and a

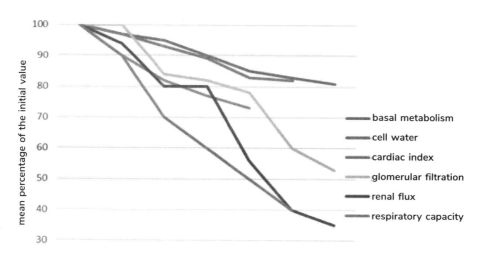

Figure 24. Modification of physiological parameters with age. On the vertical axis, mean percentage of the initial value, and on the horizontal axis, age. (See also color plate 9.)

---

2. *Homeostasis* is the word that is commonly used to refer to the balance of the functions and states of the organism. Our body seeks to maintain a relative constancy in its processes and functions. Maintaining a relatively stable heart rate or a stable body temperature are manifestations of homeostasis.

complex adaptation to a changing environment that has also required a high degree of variation in behaviors, genetic expression, and metabolic functions. If we had prioritized rigidity over homeostasis, we would have been less able to adapt to a changing environment and, conversely, internal homeostasis simply cannot be dispensed with, as it is an essential requirement for any minimally complex organism. In this complicated equation balancing flexible adaptation and maintaining homeostasis, there is no room (or need) to ensure a long life for a particular organism. We are made to adapt, not be immortal. All cells in our body, except cancer cells, are destined to die. To put it simply, over the years, more and more flaws are produced and accumulated at different levels of biological complexity. Our organs begin to fail and chronic or neurodegenerative diseases appear until we irremediably cease to exist. Evolution's only consolation (and ours as well) is having kept us alive long enough to have fulfilled our dreams, marveled at existence, made the people around us happy, and perpetuated our species. But that is up to each one of us (yes, it may be a waste of your time to be reading this book; I won't be the one to stop you if you want to throw it away and dedicate your time to more important things!).

Main Centers and Enzymes Responsible for Metabolism

Broadly speaking, this complex metabolic process takes place in two phases. A first phase consists of the oxidation, reduction, or hydrolysis of a molecule. The activity of cytochrome P450, abbreviated as CYP, also takes place in this phase. CYPs are a superfamily of proteins assigned to carry out most of the metabolic process on xenobiotics. They are found especially in the liver and there are literally dozens of different enzymes, with greater or lesser affinity for the different molecules to which they are exposed. Related to the previous point, it should be noted that CYPs perform their function progressively less effectively as we age.

In the context of CYPs, drugs or xenobiotics are classified into substrates (which "occupy" some of these enzymes, because they have an affinity for them), inducers (which enhance the activity of certain enzymes, therefore increasing their metabolic functions and processing drugs more quickly), or inhibitors (which, on the contrary, reduce the activity of certain enzymes and expose the body to potential toxic effects, since they are not able to process certain xenobiotics). Table 8 lists some psychedelics that act as substrates and inhibitors of certain CYP enzymes.

CYPs are named with the root "CYP" followed by a number designating the family to which it belongs, a letter denoting the subfamily, and another number designating the CYP form. Therefore, CYP2D6 is family 2, subfamily D, and gene number 6.

TABLE 8. EXAMPLES OF LIVER ENZYMES THAT PROCESS PSYCHEDELIC DRUGS*

	LSD	DMT	Ibogaine	Ketamine	MDMA
CYP2D6	-	Substrate	Substrate and inhibitor	-	Substrate and inhibitor
CYP3A4	Substrate	Substrate	-	Substrate	-
CYP2C19	Substrate	-	-	-	-
CYP1A2	-	-	-	-	Substrate

*In the case of substrates, it must be assumed that the metabolism of other drugs or substances that are ingested and also processed by the same enzymes will be less effective, with the consequent risk of intoxication. In the case of substances that also act as enzyme inhibitors, such as MDMA or ibogaine, this risk will be even higher.

In a second phase of metabolism, a process called conjugation takes place. It is at this time that the metabolites or substances generated by the first phase of metabolism are collected and combined with other molecules. Although the main metabolic center of our body is the liver, other organs (such as the gastrointestinal tract, the kidneys, and the lungs) also perform very important metabolic functions, especially when certain routes of administration are used.

RELEVANT ASPECTS IN THE METABOLISM OF PSYCHEDELIC DRUGS

Due to its importance and the amount of associated information, in this section we will discuss the metabolism of certain psychedelic drugs in detail. We cannot mention all the drugs that we have included in other sections of this book simply for lack of available information, since the pharmacokinetic studies necessary for the description of this process have not been carried out in all of them.

Psilocybin

As we have observed before, the metabolism and general kinetics of psilocybin are still largely unknown. We know that it quickly converts into psilocin (a fraction of psilocybin will have already undergone this transformation even before reaching the liver), surely due to the similarity of the molecule with serotonin, an amine that our body metabolizes very easily and in different organs and tissues. Psilocin is in turn metabolized in the liver, both by MAO and by aldehyde dehydrogenase enzymes, also involved in alcohol metabolism.

Disulfiram (brand name Antabuse) is a drug that inhibits these enzymes, and for this reason it is prescribed in patients with alcoholism, since by inhibiting the metabolism of alcohol severe intoxication symptoms are induced when ingested, which in theory causes aversion.

To lengthen or enhance the effects of psilocybin mushrooms, users sometimes use MAO inhibitors, although MAO inhibitors have also been identified in the mushrooms themselves, so caution should be exercised when combining these inhibitors. Tobacco is also a known

MAO inhibitor, and in fact it has been reported that regular smokers have up to 40 percent lower MAO concentrations than nonsmokers, so they would also be more likely to experience the psychoactive effects of psilocybin with greater intensity, since in any case the metabolism of psilocin would be inhibited.

The half-life of psilocin is approximately three hours in adults. In samples obtained after five hours of mushroom ingestion, it has been observed that 80 percent of the psilocin has already passed through the second phase of metabolism (conjugation of the hydrolyzed group of psilocin) and is subsequently eliminated in the urine. In fact, as we've said, this metabolic process is identical to that of serotonin.

DMT/Ayahuasca

One of the most complex and mysterious metabolisms of psychedelics is that of ayahuasca. We say mysterious because it is still not very well known how the combination or combinations of plants that allow the intense effects of this drink to unfold were originally identified by the Indigenous populations of the Amazon. As has already been said, there are many plants that inhibit human metabolism in many different ways, and there are also many plants that contain DMT. Effectively combining a plant that specifically inhibits MAO and another that contains high concentrations of DMT, and cooking them appropriately, is something that escapes any probabilistic model, also taking into account the tremendous plant diversity in the Amazon. It is also true that various systems of traditional medicine that have used plants for centuries or millennia, such as traditional Chinese medicine, have been based on the use of complex plant combinations, surely looking for ways to enhance their effects in order to have more effective remedies. In this sense, it can be assumed that the Amazonian Indigenous people also developed the strategy of combining different plants to make preparations, infusions, ointments, and the like. In this case, perhaps with the purpose of communicating with the gods, predicting the future, hunting, or simply generating more community cohesion through collective ceremonies, highly effective remedies, such as ayahuasca, could have been developed.

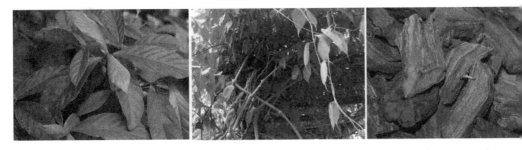

Figure 25. *Mimosa hostilis* (*left* image) and *Banisteriopsis caapi* (*center* and *right* images), plants used for ayahuasca decocting. The *M. hostilis* is rich in DMT, which, if ingested orally, would have no effect, due to the metabolism produced by monoamine oxidase (MAO). The joint decoction of this plant with the *B. caapi* vine (which contains MAO inhibitors) allows DMT not to degrade so quickly, enabling access to the central nervous system, where it deploys its particular psychoactive effects, thus constituting the complicated metabolism of ayahuasca. Original image from the article: Brito-da-Costa AM, Dias-da-Silva D, Gomes N, Dinis-Oliveira RJ, Madureira-Carvalho Á. 2020. Toxicokinetics and toxicodynamics of ayahuasca alkaloids N,N-dimethyltryptamine (DMT), harmine, harmaline and tetrahydroharmine: clinical and forensic impact. Pharmaceuticals (Basel, Switzerland) 13(11):334. Reproduced with the authors' permission. (See also color plate 8.)

The "activation" of DMT by inhibiting MAO could actually be optional if DMT was administered intravenously, since by this route we also manage to avoid metabolism, making it easier for DMT to reach the brain. However, taking it orally with MAO inhibitors has some advantages. First, the effects last longer (three to five hours) than if given intravenously (fifteen to twenty minutes), although depending on the purpose for which it is consumed, this could be seen as a disadvantage. Also the possible adverse effects related to the cardiovascular system are more tolerable, since it has been observed that the increase in blood pressure and heart rate are more subtle in the case of ayahuasca, compared to intravenous DMT.

It is worth mentioning that the absorption of ayahuasca, both of DMT and beta-carbolines, already starts in the mucosa of the mouth. Recent studies have found that the residues that remain in

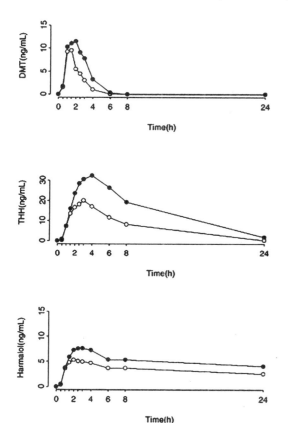

Figure 26. Measurement of blood concentrations of DMT (*top*), tetrahydroharmine (THH; *center*), and harmalol (*bottom*), in a period of twenty-four hours, after the oral administration of ayahuasca. Original image from the article: Riba J, Valle M, Urbano G, Yritia M, Morte A, Barbanoj MJ. 2003. Human pharmacology of ayahuasca: subjective and cardiovascular effects, monoamine metabolite excretion, and pharmacokinetics. The Journal of Pharmacology and Experimental Therapeutics 306(1):73–83.

the mouth after oral intake are rapidly absorbed through saliva and appear almost instantly in the bloodstream, although at very low concentrations. In fact, the maximum concentration in the bloodstream of most of the compounds of ayahuasca is reached one hour after oral intake, with the exception of tetrahydroharmine (THH), which reaches its maximum concentration two hours after ingestion. It is also the substance that takes the longest to be eliminated (more than twenty-four hours after ingestion). The half-life of DMT is just over an hour, and it almost completely disappears from the bloodstream six to eight hours after ingestion. The rest of the beta-carbolines are eliminated in the same way at around eight hours, with the exception, apart from the above-mentioned THH, of a metabolite of harmaline, harmalol, which also lasts longer than twenty-four hours after ingestion. The most important liver enzymes for the metabolism of beta-carbolines are CYP2D6 and CYP1A1, and CYP2D6 and CYP3A4 for the metabolism of DMT.

LSD

The half-life of LSD ranges between approximately 2 and 3 hours, reaching the highest peak concentration in plasma at 1.5 hours after sublingual administration. At doses of 100 micrograms, a large part of LSD has already been eliminated from the body after 12 to 14 hours, while after ingesting doses of 200 micrograms or more, this process can take up to 16 or 17 hours. The time to onset of effects can be up to 45–50 minutes after a 100-microgram dose and shortens considerably after higher doses. Interestingly, even if LSD is administered intravenously, the maximum point of subjective effects is not reached until after half an hour, although the first effects do appear in a matter of minutes. This shows an opposite effect to what happens with other similar substances, such as DMT, which reaches the peak of its effects in a matter of minutes after intravenous administration. It's not entirely clear why LSD takes so long to unfold its full effects even intravenously, but it may be that it crosses the blood-brain barrier slowly or that the chemical cascades responsible for its effects simply take time to unfold completely.

The metabolism to which LSD is exposed when entering the body is very extensive. It is estimated that only about 1 percent of the ingested dose passes directly into the urine without undergoing any alteration. This metabolism occurs primarily in the liver, where it is passed through various enzymes (CYP3A4, CYP1A2, CYP2E1, and CYP2C19) producing multiple nonpsychoactive metabolites. The analysis of metabolites and traces of LSD in urine cannot always be detected, since this is a substance that is consumed in doses of micrograms, and therefore its metabolic products are formed at even smaller doses (sub-ng/mL). Whether or not they can be detected will depend on the type of technique used, the time of sample collection, or the dose ingested, among other factors.

MDMA

We have already commented on some interesting aspects of the metabolism of MDMA, especially in relation to the increase in toxicity associated with it. It should also be noted that MDMA will be metabolized mainly in the liver in two different stages, in which MDA and other metabolites are formed. The enzymes most involved in this process are CYP2D6 and CYP1A2. Approximately two hours after administration is when the peak of the highest plasma concentration of MDMA is reached, with a half-life of about eight hours.

It has been suggested that MDMA exhibits nonlinear kinetics. We speak of nonlinear kinetics when there are unpredictable or disproportionate changes in the pharmacokinetic parameters of a substance in relation to its dose or concentration. For example, what is expected in any substance is that when the administered dose is increased, the concentrations of the substance in plasma, for example, also proportionally increase. When this is not the case, the substance is said to have nonlinear kinetics. This type of kinetics generally occurs due to saturation of the metabolism centers, due to saturation of protein binding, or due to inadequate renal transport of the substance, causing it to accumulate and making the concentrations that reach the liver and kidney greater than those that can be eliminated. This is what happens in the case of MDMA, and specifically it appears that MDMA metabolites bind to and inhibit the CYP2D6 enzyme, making its metabolism much less effective.

The inhibition of CYP2D6 by the metabolites of MDMA lasts longer than twenty-four hours, so caution should also be exercised when consuming other substances or medications during this period, as the user will be exposed to potential intoxications and suffer more side effects.

It is estimated that 30 percent of all current drugs are metabolized by CYP2D6. In this way, it can be said that MDMA inhibits its own metabolism, and for this reason redosing is so dangerous, because if more MDMA is consumed while under its effects, there is a greater risk of intoxication since its metabolism will be inhibited. This means that an additional dose of just 40 mg can have the same effects as a dose of 80 mg or more, so repeated dosing should always be avoided and, if doing so, doses should be very, very low.

Mescaline

The half-life of mescaline is about six hours. Most of the metabolism will be carried out by the liver and kidneys. Interestingly, the peak of psychological effects of mescaline (approximately two hours) may not coincide with the peak of mescaline concentrations in the brain. In fact, it has been suggested that some metabolites of mescaline may be widely involved in the psychoactive effects experienced after ingestion; yet there are still no studies that have been able to clarify these unknowns. We do not even know whether this first metabolism, that supposedly generates a psychoactive metabolite, is carried out by MAO or by diamine oxidase (DAO). This scenario is already complicated, considering the administration of pure mescaline, but it becomes much more complicated if we consider the use of peyote or San Pedro preparations, since it has been hypothesized that these contain other psychoactive compounds, which could play an additional role in the development of its psychological effects.

Ketamine

Ketamine metabolism also occurs primarily in the liver, by the enzyme CYP3A4 and others to a lesser extent. One of the ketamine metabolites, norketamine, is also psychoactive and has anesthetic and analgesic properties, so it is possible to report therapeutic effects even when ketamine has already stopped working. Ketamine has fairly rapid kinetics, with a half-life of two to four hours, which is partly why it has been widely used as an anesthetic.

The enantiomers (S)- and (R)-ketamine also have very short half-lives (approximately 1.5 hours). (S)-ketamine is twice as potent as ketamine, and about 4 times as potent as (R)-ketamine. In fact, intravenous anesthesia requires a dose of 275 mg of ketamine, 430 mg of (R)-ketamine, and 140 mg of (S)-ketamine. Ketamine and its metabolites are excreted via the kidneys, with only 2 percent of the ketamine dose remaining unchanged.

Ibogaine/Noribogaine

Ibogaine metabolism not only plays an important role in its processing and subsequent elimination from the body, but is also crucial for its antiaddictive effects. In animal models, it has been observed that, with the reduction of first-pass metabolism, for example, by administering ibogaine intravenously or subcutaneously, such drastic reductions in withdrawal symptoms associated with drugs of abuse are not observed. Since its main metabolite, noribogaine, is produced in the metabolism of ibogaine, these findings demonstrate the important role of noribogaine in the therapeutic effects of ibogaine. Although it surely must be a combination of the effects of both substances, since ibogaine cannot be considered a prodrug.

In the metabolism of ibogaine, specifically in its absorption and elimination, nonlinear kinetics have also been observed, so, again, this suggests caution when using repeated doses, as toxic concentrations can easily be reached. The reasons for the possible saturation when processing ibogaine are diverse. First, it is a substance that is metabolized slowly, due to its structural complexity, which is why liver enzymes are less efficient in metabolizing this substance compared to others. Second, ibogaine and noribogaine produce what is called enterohepatic circulation. That is, they pass through the liver, are metabolized, transported to the bile, which carries them to the intestine, and there they are again transported back to the liver to start the whole process again (see figure 27). This prolongs the action of both substances, although mainly of noribogaine, and also saturates the metabolism of ibogaine as it cannot effectively eliminate the substances that have already been metabolized. Finally, parallel to this process, we must remember that both substances, ibogaine and noribogaine, are widely fat soluble, so they will bind to a large amount of fat in our body, releasing slowly and continuously for

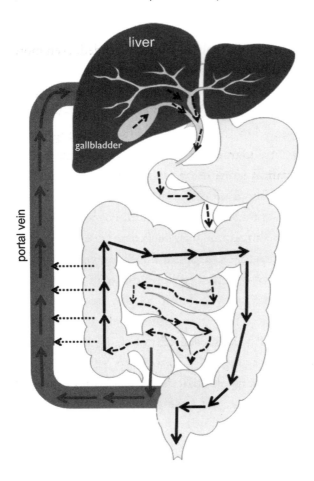

Figure 27. Enterohepatic circulation. In the case of ibogaine, this substance and its main metabolite, noribogaine, leave the liver and pass through the intestine, where part of them is again transported through the hepatic portal vein to the liver, where they will be processed and metabolized again.

hours and, in the case of noribogaine, days. Consequently, in the case of using repeated doses of ibogaine, the metabolism will be continuously saturated, not only by the concentrations of the first dose and additional doses, but also by the amounts of both substances stored in adipose tissue, which are continuously released in the bloodstream.

The most important hepatic enzyme in the metabolism of ibogaine is CYP2D6. There are few data on the kinetics of ibogaine, and the only ones obtained in the context of a controlled clinical trial were obtained after administering a very low dose (20 mg). In that study, a half-life of two to five hours was observed for ibogaine, and about thirteen hours for noribogaine. When the dose of ibogaine is much higher, as is often the case in therapeutic contexts (in which doses of more than 1 g can be reached), it is expected that the half-life times will be extended, even more so knowing the nonlinear kinetics of the substance. In the same study, the CYP2D6 enzyme was also inhibited in a small sample of healthy volunteers by administering paroxetine, a potent inhibitor. They received the same 20-mg dose of ibogaine, but the half-lives were much longer (ten hours for ibogaine and twenty hours for noribogaine). We must assume that the half-lives of near-gram doses of ibogaine should be closer to these numbers, although future studies will need to assess the kinetics of therapeutic doses of ibogaine. It should be noted that when noribogaine is administered directly, its half-life is remarkably longer (twenty-eight to forty-nine hours), so its safety profile is a priori more unfavorable than if the substance is produced as a result of ibogaine metabolism.

Salvinorin-A

Salvinorin-A has to be absorbed through saliva by chewing *S. divinorum* leaves or, ideally, via the lungs through vaporization, to prevent its rapid metabolism. In fact, when it enters the bloodstream, it is metabolized by blood esterases, mainly adding hydroxyl groups to the molecule (making it more soluble in water). Therefore, it would be necessary to consume a huge amount of salvinorin-A orally so that even after going through first-pass metabolism and metabolism by blood esterases, we would still be left with a sufficient concentration to cross the blood-brain barrier and unfold its effects. It is also extensively processed by different enzymes in the liver: CYP2D6, CYP2C18, CYP1A1, and CYP2E1. After passing through these enzymes, salvinorin-B, its main metabolite, is produced. However, this does not seem to reach relevant concentrations in plasma, so it is completely inactive.

As can be inferred from the short duration of its effects, salvinorin-A exhibits very rapid kinetics, with a half-life of less than one hour. Likewise, less than 1 percent of salvinorin-A is excreted unchanged in the urine between one and two hours after inhaled consumption, which corroborates its extensive metabolism. It is estimated that there is no trace of salvinorin-A in the urine after four to six hours.

Tropane Alkaloids

All the alkaloids that we can find in plants such as *D. stramonium* are rapidly metabolized, with the exception of scopolamine. While the half-life of atropine is about two to three hours, that of scopolamine is eight hours or more. The time it takes to produce maximum effects can vary between one and three hours, although it should be noted that the route of administration is also crucial in this case.

The bioavailability of scopolamine, for example, when administered orally, is quite limited. In twenty to thirty minutes, the maximum plasma concentrations are reached and the half-life is around one hour. Due to its rapid kinetics when administered orally and the adverse effects associated with intravenous use (hallucinations, dry mouth, dizziness, to name a few), its clinical use is fairly limited to transdermal patches. These patches work as an extended release system. They are generally worn for seventy-two hours, during which time the scopolamine is slowly released. They are made up of four layers. The first layer basically consists of a polyester film with aluminum, and it is the layer that will be furthest from the skin. In the second layer we find a mixture of scopolamine, mineral oil, and other compounds that bind the mixture. The third layer contains a polypropylene membrane that controls the release of the substance. Finally, the fourth layer, and the one that will be in direct contact with the skin, is an adhesive that also contains mineral oil and a first primer of 140 micrograms of scopolamine. After application of the patch, the first plasma concentrations of scopolamine are reached at four hours, reaching the maximum concentration at twenty-four hours. The release rate of scopolamine in these patches is approximately 0.5 mg per day.

In the case of atropine, it can be administered intravenously or intramuscularly, since the maximum concentrations in plasma are reached quickly via one route or another. The half-life is around three hours, as we have said, although in elderly patients this lasts up to ten hours. There are also some gender differences. While women seem to absorb more atropine, showing higher plasma concentrations, they also eliminate it earlier, with half-life times being somewhat shorter than in men.

Both atropine and scopolamine are metabolized mainly in the liver, although between 40 and 50 percent of these are excreted unchanged in the urine. The enzymes responsible for its metabolism are CYP2C9, CYP2D6, and CYP3A4, among others with less relevance.

ELIMINATION

This last phase of metabolism is perhaps the least complex in terms of the amount of information needed to understand its operation. It is basically a matter of identifying the routes of drug excretion.

We have already seen in previous sections that the drugs or substances that are ingested can be eliminated, either without alterations or as metabolites. We have also seen that polar (water soluble) substances are eliminated more easily than nonpolar (lipid soluble) substances. In fact, one of the main functions of metabolism is to make the latter compounds more water soluble to facilitate their elimination.

In the excretion of xenobiotics in general, the kidney is the most important organ, since up to 30 percent of marketed drugs will be eliminated unchanged via this route, in addition to the metabolites, bile, or other products resulting from their metabolism. Drugs or other substances are also eliminated via other routes, such as breast milk, and, although in this case the concentration of substances or metabolites excreted is very low, it may be relevant for possible effects on an infant. Likewise, it is necessary to consider age as one of the factors that will affect the elimination of xenobiotics, since renal function deteriorates approximately 1 percent per year after maturity has been reached (thirty to thirty-five years); therefore, in elderly people the elimination process will be carried out in a progressively less efficient way.

There are a few relevant aspects to comment on regarding the elimination profiles of most psychedelic drugs, so we will summarize them in the following paragraphs. In the case of psilocybin, as we have seen, it is rapidly eliminated, and it is already undetectable in urine in twenty-four hours. Two to six hours after ingestion is when more psilocin is eliminated in the urine.

Ayahuasca is somewhat more complex, as can be deduced. On the one hand, it is necessary to analyze the excretion of DMT and, on the other, that of beta-carbolines. The first undergoes extensive metabolism that ends up excreting less than 1 percent of the initial dose unchanged in the urine, as well as significant quantities of some of its metabolites, such as DMT-N-oxide. The moment in which the greatest excretion of DMT and its metabolites occurs postingestion is after two hours and up to seven to eight hours.

The beta-carbolines and their metabolites also undergo extensive metabolism, especially harmine. However, they are eliminated in a more spaced manner for twenty-four hours after, and in the case of some metabolites, they are still found in the urine two and three days after ingesting ayahuasca. In the first eight hours after ingestion, about 50 percent of harmine has already been excreted. In contrast, only 30 percent of harmaline and THH have been excreted in this time frame, showing slower metabolism and elimination.

As already mentioned, LSD is rapidly metabolized and converted into different metabolites. The greatest excretion of these substances in the urine takes place four to six hours after administration. Progressively more concentrations of these metabolites are excreted, which are still detectable four days after taking 200 micrograms. Unchanged LSD, on the other hand, is only detectable up to 30 hours after ingestion of 100 micrograms. If the dose is doubled, five more hours are added to this period: 35 hours after consuming 200 micrograms, 40 hours after consuming 400 micrograms, and so on.

MDMA has fairly slow elimination kinetics. After administration of a low dose of MDMA (1 mg/kg), it can be detected unchanged in the urine up to one hundred forty hours after consumption, and its metabolites up to one hundred forty-two hours. After a high dose (1.6 mg/kg), unchanged MDMA can be detected up to one hundred forty-nine hours after consumption and its metabolites (especially HMMA) up to one hundred sixty hours. It should be noted that MDMA is one of the substances that is excreted in breast milk, so it is advisable not to breast-feed if it has been consumed for at least the next two hundred hours, for safety reasons. Tropane alkaloids such as atropine and scopolamine are also excreted in breast milk.

The reader will also remember that mescaline has very poor absorption. This means that a high percentage of consumed mescaline is excreted unchanged in urine. Indeed, around 80 percent of consumed mescaline is eliminated in the urine after the first hour of ingestion, and 13 percent in the form of a metabolite (TMPA). This metabolite is progressively eliminated while the mescaline that has been absorbed is metabolized, and it is detectable up to seventy-two hours after consumption.

Ketamine also undergoes intense metabolism and we will only find 2 percent of the unchanged dose of ketamine in urine. Most of its metabolites are hydrolyzed ketamine compounds. Repeated doses of ketamine can accumulate and extend its complete elimination up to eleven days. On the other hand, some of its metabolites, such as norketamine, can be found in the urine up to fourteen days after a single administration of ketamine. After administration of a single dose of ketamine, most of it has been eliminated after twelve hours. This could partly explain the prolonged efficacy of ketamine treatments for depression, although their effects on some markers of neuroplasticity are also implicated. In the case of ketamine, a relevant aspect to take into account, and one that does not occur in other psychedelic drugs, is the toxicity to the urinary tract. It appears that the contact of ketamine and its metabolites with the mucosa of the urinary tract could be toxic and cause some serious adverse effects such as bladder irritation or cystitis. Another possibility that has been raised is that ketamine could alter the permeability between urine and bladder tissues, causing toxic substances present in urine to access the bladder wall, causing structural damage or possible infection. Although interstitial fibrosis, chronic renal failure, and other associated problems have been reported in chronic users of high doses of ketamine, it seems that the administration of occasional doses as treatment for depression would be safe.

It has also been previously mentioned that the liver is mainly responsible for the metabolism of ibogaine. However, it seems that the biliary and gastrointestinal routes prevail for its elimination.

Ninety percent of a high dose (20 mg/kg) of ibogaine is eliminated within twenty-four hours, whereas noribogaine is eliminated much more slowly, and plasma concentrations can be found even four to five days after intake. This occurs on the one hand due to the high lipophilic profile of both substances, which causes them to bind to fatty tissue and be gradually released through enterohepatic circulation, and on the other to the metabolic saturation that is typically caused by substances with nonlinear kinetics, as the reader may already know.

Finally, the elimination of salvinorin-A occurs mainly via the kidneys in the case of the hydrolyzed metabolites and also through the bile, in the case of the more fat-soluble metabolites. Salvinorin-A is rapidly eliminated from the body, consistent with its rapid kinetics. After inhalation of a high dose (1 mg), a half-life of about fifty minutes was reported in a study. In another less controlled study, where dried leaves of *S. divinorum* were consumed, only 0.8 percent of pure salvinorin-A was found in the urine, completely disappearing after one and a half hours.

TABLE 9. ELIMINATION TIMES OF THE MAIN PSYCHEDELIC DRUGS FROM THE BODY*

Complete elimination times of the organism	
Salvinorin-A	1.5 hours
DMT	8 hours
Ketamine	12 hours
Ibogaine	24 hours
Psilocybin	24 hours
LSD	30 hours
Beta-carbolines	3 days
Noribogaine	5 days
MDMA	149 hours

*These are the mean elimination times after urinalysis, which does not imply that the elimination times may not vary by individual. In addition, other methods can still find traces of these substances or their metabolites long after, such as in the analysis of hair samples.

Pharmacodynamics

Having examined pharmacokinetics, we will now look at pharmacodynamics, which is the study of the biochemical or physiological effects of drugs or substances, as well as their mechanisms of action. Chapter 3 of this book has already described the main targets of the most representative psychedelic drugs, at least in the field of cellular receptors. Therefore, the binding profile to these receptors will not be described again here; only in some cases will this information be expanded by adding certain specific targets or commenting on their specific effects, for example on hormones and brain regions. Instead of focusing on the mechanisms of action, we will deal directly with the results of their interaction, talking about their therapeutic effects, adverse effects, and psychoactive effects.

In the field of psychedelic research, when we study pharmacodynamics we do not limit ourselves to cellular or physiological effects. Instead, a vast realm of psychoactive effects opens up for us to describe. This description has been quite limited in the history of pharmacology, not only because of the small number of drugs and natural products that are capable of altering our perceptual functions compared to those that cannot, but also because their study has not enjoyed adequate complexity or richness until relatively recently. Of course, Louis Lewin (German pharmacologist and pioneer of psychoactive research, 1850–1929) and Moreau de Tours, among many other later authors, systematically studied the effects of some psychedelic drugs, but it was not until a few years ago that studies began using standardized tools or correlating subjective phenomena with objective neuroimaging measurements, hormone levels, or pharmacokinetic parameters, which have undoubtedly taken the study of psychoactive effects to a higher level.

From the point of view of pharmacodynamics, psychedelic drugs also possess a small peculiarity that, at the very least, invites philosophical reflection. Traditionally in pharmacology, it is understood that the effects produced by drugs only alter the speed or magnitude of intrinsic cellular responses, instead of creating new responses. If we follow this definition in the case of psychedelic drugs, we may conclude either that their profound effects on consciousness and perception of internal and external reality are only more dramatic alterations of functions that certain chemicals are already performing in our body or that instead of producing strange effects that should not occur under normal conditions, they present these cellular and biochemical responses that modulate the perception of reality as a natural occurrence. In fact, you only need to think about the effects associated with oxytocin (trust, love, emotional bonds) or cortisol (alertness, fear) to become aware of the dramatic alterations of reality that certain substances can cause.

Before we get started describing the pharmacodynamics of psychedelic drugs, it should be noted that there is a wide variability in the response to drugs or substances in general, but even more so in the case of psychedelics, since their effects will depend on a great number of factors. In the case of nonpsychoactive drugs, the response to them may vary between different people due to factors such as the presence of diseases, age, diet, and lifestyle, but also within the same person due, for example, to biochemical or hematological alterations, tolerance, water consumption, time of day, or season of the year in which the medicine is taken. However, in the case of psychoactive drugs or substances, the psychological experience will vary. First of all, no two psychological experiences are ever the same (each time we visit an amusement park, for example, we have a different experience, which is why we go repeatedly and gladly pay for tickets again), but also because our emotional state, mood, or our economic or social circumstances, as well as the contexts in which the substance is consumed, will not be the same, all producing a unique and unrepeatable experience. Hence, no predictions can be made about the experience that an active dose of psilocybin or LSD will produce in an individual. This means that in this section we are going to describe general effects, which tend to occur quite frequently, and also some that may not occur as often, but in any case we must keep in mind at all times the great variability of effects and not assume any of the information that is going to be presented below as absolute truth, but rather as tendencies or approximations of a highly complex phenomenon.

THERAPEUTIC EFFECTS OF PSYCHEDELICS

When we looked at the pharmacological targets of psychedelics, we mentioned that almost all of them share a distinctive characteristic: the activation of the 5-HT2A subreceptor. An important part of their therapeutic effects can be explained by their action on this specific receptor and on the serotonin neurotransmission system in general. However, it is advisable not to fall into myopic views and exclude other mechanisms. A recent study,[3] for example, showed that psilocybin has antidepressant properties independent of the 5-HT2A receptor, which suggests that its action on this receptor may not be the only clinically useful one. In addition, if we bypass the 5-HT2A agonism, we will also prevent the psychedelic effects from unfolding, and this will necessarily result in a higher safety profile and in many more people willing to go through these treatments. It must be admitted, despite certain romantic arguments and discourses in favor of psychedelia, that it is a minority of the population that would be willing to take psychedelic drugs, whatever the context, and comparatively close to a majority (in reference to the general population) that are suffering the devastating consequences of mental disorders. Consequently, it is more necessary than ever to investigate mechanisms of action independent of the 5-HT2A receptor.

With that in mind, the history of psychopharmacological research on depression is unfortunate and, ironically, depressing. It is a story of constant setbacks, conflicts of interest, and many deaths along the way. Rational drug design requires minimal knowledge of the pathophysiology of a given disease in order to design or select drugs that can

3. Hesselgrave N, Troppoli TA, Wulff AB, Cole AB, Thompson SM. 2021. Harnessing psilocybin: antidepressant-like behavioral and synaptic actions of psilocybin are independent of 5-HT2R activation in mice. Proceedings of the National Academy of Sciences of the United States of America 118(17):e2022489118.

correct it. However, when the monoaminergic hypothesis of depression prevailed,[4] the efficacy of antidepressant drugs was explained by the increase of monoamines in the synaptic space. When this hypothesis was no longer popular, their efficacy began to be explained by the ability of many antidepressants to induce neuroplasticity. Both views lacked solid evidence that these drugs actually work or are better than a placebo. This is due to many factors, but luckily, we are already nearing another stage in psychopharmacology, and reductionist approaches are becoming less predominant and more questionable.

There is another aspect we must address when considering the potential beneficial effects of psychedelics, and that is that the way to demonstrate their usefulness is through clinical trials. We must be aware that despite being considered the "gold standard" in clinical research, clinical trials have their limitations. The esteemed pharmacologist and father of current pharmacovigilance in Europe, Joan-Ramon Laporte, states the following about clinical trials:

> In a therapeutic clinical trial, a comparison is made, and the key question is to determine whether there are differences between the compared interventions to make patients in health state A transition (or not) to a new more favorable state B. The fact that the intervention precedes in time to state B does not necessarily imply that the intervention is the cause of B. To draw this conclusion would be to commit the *post hoc ergo propter hoc* fallacy.
>
> In clinical trials, as in biology in general, one cannot speak of unicausal and unequivocal relationships between causes and effects. Instead, the notion of contributory cause is used. . . .
>
> However, due to interindividual variability, it is often not possible to isolate a single variable and study it individually, so that in biology the contributory cause is identified as an average value. Thus, not all patients subjected to a contributory cause will manifest the

---

4. The monoaminergic hypothesis, as its name indicates, consisted of explaining the pathology of depression as a deficit in the concentrations of a particular amine, serotonin.

expected effect, or in other words, not all patients treated with a "proven effective" drug will respond favorably to its administration.

Therefore, if a clinical trial with a psychedelic yields some benefit, the most we can say based on the evidence is that the psychedelic in question will be a possible contributory cause and, certainly, we cannot affirm that all people exposed to that psychedelic will respond in the same way. Laporte continues:

> It is not always possible to assume that the results obtained in the context of a clinical trial can be extrapolated to the conditions of regular practice. Thus, for example, the results obtained with a new surgical technique in a clinical trial cannot be directly extrapolated to regular practice in other centers that did not participate in the trial, because the surgeon is not the same, nor is the quality of the nursing service, the treated populations, etc. The same happens with drugs, because the conditions of a clinical trial (participating centers, type of relationship with patients, diagnostic criteria applied, clinical supervision, etc.) are not the same as in regular practice.[5]

This is a fundamental factor to consider in the case of psychedelics. The framework in which most studies are conducted is as ideal as it is illusory. Suddenly, people who are included in clinical trials move from the overwhelmed public health systems, where they are lucky if someone attends to them once a month to prescribe some drug, to enjoying twenty-four-hour care with a team of the country's best professionals and therapists who genuinely care for their health, perform a multitude of tests for free, and also spend long experimental sessions with them in which they can discuss aspects of their life and the most relevant conflicts. The benefits that this therapeutic context will have for the individual are unlikely to occur in regular clinical practice, where, although

---

5. Laporte JR. 1993. Principios básicos de investigación clínica [Basic principles of clinical investigation]. Madrid (Spain): Ergón. Spanish.

a psychedelic may be administered when these treatments are approved in the future, the rest of the conditions will continue to be lamentable and precarious.

Antidepressant, Anti-inflammatory, and Neuroprotective Effects

After the cautionary note above, we can now focus on the effects directly associated with the agonism of psychedelics on the 5-HT2A receptor. For starters, we can mention that the interaction with this receptor causes antidepressant, anti-inflammatory, and neuroprotective effects, although these effects should not be seen separately, since inflammatory processes, for example, are closely related to depression, so if we induce an anti-inflammatory effect, we will also partially obtain an antidepressant effect; the same thing happens in the case of neuroprotection.

Regarding antidepressant effects, we must mention that the brain regions with the highest density of the 5-HT2A receptor are the prefrontal cortex (PFC); the cortices of the parietal, temporal, and occipital lobes; the entorhinal area; certain nuclei of the hypothalamus; the claustrum; and the lateral nuclei of the amygdala. These regions are involved in many cognitive processes, emotional regulation, introspection, and self-awareness, among others, so, in a nutshell, with the modulation of all these functions we can "improve someone's mood," as it is popularly referred to. This is achieved in different ways, both from a production increase and release of serotonin, as well as glutamate neurotransmission, which ends up generating neuroplasticity, a phenomenon that we will deal with in depth later, and which has also been associated with antidepressant effects.

Regarding anti-inflammatory effects, although serotonin is often involved in inflammatory processes, interestingly, activation of its receptors by psychedelics has been associated with potent anti-inflammatory effects. This was discovered relatively recently, in 2008, when it was observed that LSD and other psychedelics, but especially 2,5-dimethoxy-4-iodoamphetamine (DOI), a compound of the phenethylamine family, very potently inhibited all markers of inflammation associated with tumor necrosis factor (TNF), a cytokine[6] produced in immune cells causing inflammation and cell death. When psychedelics are administered together with selective 5-HT2A receptor antagonists, the anti-inflammatory effect disappears. These extraordinary effects are being studied for diseases that go beyond mental health, since inflammatory processes are related to many diseases. Specifically, studies are being conducted for the treatment of asthma, atherosclerosis, and inflammatory bowel disease with 5-HT2A agonists derived from DOI (or other psychedelics). It should be noted that, at least in studies with animal models, the doses of DOI required to produce therapeutic effects were much lower than those required to produce behavioral changes.

The last of the effects associated with the stimulation of the 5-HT2A receptor is that of neuroprotection. Substances with a neuroprotective effect are all those that protect neurons from toxic metabolic products or from diseases or conditions associated with the loss of or damage to neuronal bodies. The very functions of brain biochemistry produce neurotoxicity. This is due to the presence of stress and subsequent release of free radicals or oxidation processes, for example, when MAO degrades amines (which is why MAO inhibitors generally have a neuroprotective effect, because by interrupting this oxidation they stop releasing neurotoxic substances). These neurotoxic effects are well tolerated most of the time, although damage can accumulate over the years and, needless to say, the brain is progressively less resilient to the neurotoxicity associated with its own functioning, so wear and tear is increasing and is what, in advanced age, ends up producing some symptoms of cognitive deterioration.

Stimulation of the 5-HT2A subreceptor appears to protect against some of the effects associated with neurotoxicity. For example, mitochondrial biogenesis is promoted, a phenomenon that renews and strengthens the function of the mitochondria. When dysfunctions occur in the mitochondria, it produces oxidative stress reactions, closely

---

6. Immune proteins that fulfill different functions, mainly inducing inflammation in the face of possible threats.

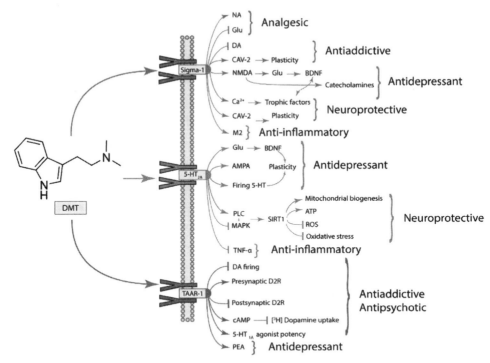

Figure 28. Main mechanisms of action by which DMT exerts analgesic, antiaddictive, antidepressant, neuroprotective, anti-inflammatory, and antipsychotic effects. Original image from the article: Ona G, Bouso JC. 2021. Therapeutic potential of natural psychoactive drugs for central nervous system disorders: a perspective from polypharmacology. Current Medicinal Chemistry 28(1):53–68. Reproduced with the authors' permission.
(See also color plate 10.)

related, for example, to aging and to cardiovascular, neurological, and metabolic diseases, as well as cancer, among others. When we engage in moderate exercise regularly, or after the consumption of large amounts of polyphenols through our diet, mitochondrial biogenesis is also enhanced. Thus, after 5-HT2A stimulation, we can prevent the release of reactive oxygen species and the appearance of the cascades that produce neurotoxicity through oxidative stress.

In addition to 5-HT2A, the action of psychedelics on other receptors can also produce antidepressant, anti-inflammatory, or neuroprotective effects. In the case of DMT, for example, its agonism on the receptor sigma-1 is associated with antidepressant effects thanks to the release of neurotrophic factors (such as BDNF)[7] and to the production of catecholamines such as adrenaline or noradrenaline, as well as having powerful anti-inflammatory effects. When DMT is consumed through ayahuasca, we will not only obtain antidepressant, anti-inflammatory, and neuroprotective effects derived from the activation of the 5-HT2A receptor and sigma-1, but these effects will be enhanced by the antidepressant and neuroprotective effects (through MAO inhibition) associated with the beta-carbolines, and by other phenolic compounds that have been identified in ayahuasca and that also exert a powerful neuroprotective effect. It should also be noted that DMT, mescaline, or LSD activate the TAAR1 receptor, as we saw in chapter 3, which has repercussions on antidepressant effects due to the greater release of phenethylamine associated with its activation.

Therapeutic Effects of Atypical Psychedelics

We are forced to devote a small section to psychedelics that not only interact with receptors other than 5-HT2A, producing therapeutic effects, but do not even bind to 5-HT2A. This is the case with ketamine, for example, which acts primarily as an NMDA receptor antagonist. Blockade of this receptor activates serotonergic neurons in the cortex, increasing glutamate release and generating neuroplasticity through BDNF release and other pathways. In addition, similar to what happens after the activation of 5-HT2A, ketamine also improves mitochondrial biogenesis, although it has been reported that in high doses it has the opposite effect, releasing more reactive oxygen species.

Ibogaine and noribogaine do not interact in a relevant way with serotonin receptors either; however, they do interact with other receptor systems producing very interesting effects. First of all, they are mu-opioid receptor antagonists and kappa agonists. Both actions are related to drug addiction treatment and, furthermore, kappa-receptor

---

7. Neurotrophic factors are proteins directly related to the induction of neuroplasticity.

agonists have also been associated with antidepressant and neuroprotective effects. The kappa is in some ways the opposite receptor to the mu. While the agonists of the latter generate euphoria and dependence, the kappa agonists tend to generate aversion to drugs of abuse and uncomfortable and unpleasant sensations (perhaps for this reason the experience with ibogaine is very often quite heavy and challenging). It has been hypothesized that, in relation to their antiaddictive effects, ibogaine and noribogaine regulate the activity of the kappa receptor and its main endogenous ligand, dynorphin, since the "kappa-dynorphin" system is altered when there is an established addictive behavior.

Continuing with the antiaddictive effects of ibogaine, it also modulates dopaminergic and serotonergic neurotransmission, mainly through its transporters (DAT and SERT, respectively), also correcting their dysfunctions, especially in the case of drug addiction. For example, it prevents the massive release of dopamine associated with drugs of abuse, such as cocaine or amphetamine, preventing the development of addiction. Its actions on nicotinic or NMDA receptors are also directly related to its antiaddictive properties, also inducing neuroplasticity through the release of neurotrophic factors. Overall, it seems that ibogaine or one of its derivatives may be useful not only in the treatment of drug addiction but also of disorders such as PTSD or even neurodegenerative diseases such as Parkinson's disease. Future studies will have to continue investigating its therapeutic properties. Lastly, I would like to comment that when ibogaine was marketed in France under the trade name Lambarene, it listed some infectious diseases in its information leaflet. Because it is an alkaloid found in the root bark of the *T. iboga*, it is possible that it shows some antimicrobial properties, since many chemicals that are synthesized in the roots or rhizomes of plants are produced precisely to protect themselves from soil pathogens. This makes them useful for combating pathogens that attack humans as well. Although today the potential of ibogaine as an antimicrobial is unknown, perhaps in the future it may have some application in this regard.

In the case of salvinorin-A, its pharmacological peculiarities were already discussed in the previous chapter. Instead of being interesting for a possible therapeutic use, these have inspired a huge number of compounds derived from salvinorin-A for research in the treatment of pain (kappa-opioid receptor agonists generate analgesia without the euphoria and dependence associated with mu-receptor agonists), drug addiction, and depression. It has also been reported that salvinorin-A protects against neurotoxic damage in conditions of hypoxia (lack of oxygen) in the brain, and although it does not interact directly with it, its potent agonism over the kappa receptor does modulate the peripheral endocannabinoid system, which opens interesting lines of research. Apart from these possible therapeutic applications, which will necessarily be analyzed over the next few years, basically the clinical trials with salvinorin-A have served to continue investigating the nature of complex phenomena, such as hallucinations or consciousness.

Tropane alkaloids have been extensively studied and their pharmacodynamic profile is fairly well known in terms of their therapeutic effects. As for scopolamine, it is mainly used for the treatment of dizziness associated with driving, nausea, and vomiting. Its antagonistic action on muscarinic receptors induces sedative effects and relaxes the activity of the nervous system in general, relaxing the smooth muscles, thereby reducing dizziness. Regarding vomiting and nausea, scopolamine reduces them because in the medulla oblongata, the brain center of the vomiting reflex, there is a high density of muscarinic receptors; therefore, any substance that is capable of antagonizing their activity will reduce vomiting and sickness. While at therapeutic doses we find these effects, at high doses scopolamine no longer acts as a sedative, but instead induces stimulating effects, accompanied by hallucinations, amnesia, and other symptoms.

Regarding atropine, its main indication today is as a cardiotonic. Almost identically to scopolamine, atropine inhibits the parasympathetic nervous system response. This is responsible for inducing relaxation and slowing down basic functions such as heartbeat, therefore, by inhibiting the parasympathetic nervous system response, parameters such as heart rate are accelerated. Generally, when someone has fewer than forty-five to fifty beats per minute, bradycardia is considered present and, if the normal heartbeat is not restored through changes in posture or other strategies, intravenous atropine is administered.

Increased Neuroplasticity

A common feature to almost all psychedelics is their ability to induce neuroplasticity. We are specifically talking about ayahuasca, DMT and derivatives (5-MeO-DMT), ibogaine/noribogaine, psilocybin, ketamine, LSD, and others that have not been talked about as much, such as DOI.

> Scientific publications in recent years have begun calling psychedelic drugs "psychoplastogens" due to their great ability to promote brain plasticity.

These neuroplastic effects are mainly regulated by an increase in glutamate neurotransmission, which is one of the consequences of 5-HT2A receptor agonism. Part of the plasticity effects occur due to an increase in c-Fos, a protein linked to neuroplasticity, as well as neurotrophic factors. Sigma-1 receptor agonists also induce neuro-plasticity, so, in the case of ayahuasca and DMT, their action on this receptor would have an additive effect on plasticity. Ketamine induces plasticity through its antagonism on NMDA receptors, and in this case it has been reported that, in general, the plasticity it induces is less than that produced by psychedelics such as LSD or DOI. This suggests that the plasticity mediated by 5-HT2A agonism might be preferable.

But what exactly is neuroplasticity? It is often said that this concept was coined by the great Spanish scientist Ramón y Cajal, although that is not entirely true. The first known reference to the term *neuroplastic* or *plasticity*, referring to a property of the nervous system, dates back to the end of the nineteenth century, and was made by Ioan Minea, a scientist from Romania. However, although he did not invent the concept, the work of Ramón y Cajal was of fundamental importance both in subsequent research of his time and in current approaches in neuroscience. This is because, through his experiments, he was able to detect and describe the characteristic plasticity of the nervous system, despite the fact that most scientists of the time defended a completely opposite position: that we have a finite number of neurons and that the tissues of the nervous system cannot regenerate.

Neuroplasticity is often defined as the ability of the nervous system to adopt new functional or structural states in response to internal or external factors. This definition, which for all practical purposes is useless because nobody understands it (like so many other things in neuroscience), actually means that the intricate networks that make up the neuronal bodies, far from being something static, a wiring that is there to transmit nerve impulses and little else, are a living, dynamic tissue that continuously adapts to the needs of the moment to give an adequate answer and function as well as possible, with the sole intention of making the person perfectly adapted to their environment. When we talk about brain plasticity, we are actually saying that the neural circuits that form it are capable of modifying its structure or its functionality.

A classic example of neuroplasticity can be found in a study[8] of the brains of London cabbies. Over several years, not only London taxi drivers but also license applicants were studied through neuroimaging tests, comparing both groups with non-taxi drivers. These studies were able to confirm that the high memory capacity that being a taxi driver in London demanded (it requires, or required, before the introduction of GPS, the memorization of twenty-five thousand streets within a radius of about ten kilometers) increases the size of the hippocampus, the brain region highly linked to memory. In fact, the more experienced the drivers were, the more volume their

---

8. Woollett K, Spiers HJ, Maguire EA. 2009. Talent in the taxi: a model system for exploring expertise. Philosophical Transactions of the Royal Society of London. Series B, Biological Sciences 364(1522):1407–1416.

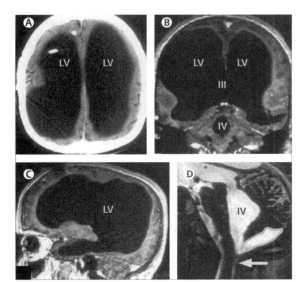

Figure 29. Brain images of a patient who, despite having only 25 percent of his brain mass, led a completely normal life. Original image from the article: Feuillet L, Dufour H, Pelletier, J. 2007. Brain of a white-collar worker. The Lancet 370(9583):262. Reproduced with the authors' permission. (See also color plate 11.)

hippocampus had. This is a fairly illustrative example of what brain plasticity means. Faced with demands from the environment but also internal ones (psychotherapy, the practice of mindfulness, and other activities have also been associated with anatomical changes in certain brain regions), our brain responds by reconfiguring its neural connections. Thus, the metaphor described by Plotinus in his Enneads is proved right. In it, he encourages us to sculpt ourselves like statues, "until the divine glory of virtue shines out on us." Well, thanks to its great plastic capacity, which even manifests itself anatomically, through our decisions, demands, and vital paths, we will be literally sculpting our brain.

Another somewhat more extreme example of neuroplasticity was published in a scientific article[9] in 2007. In it, magnetic resonance images were presented of a patient who apparently had no brain. More accurately, he only had 25 percent of his brain mass. This was due to an operation he had undergone when he was fourteen years old, and yet, despite this, he led a completely normal life without any notable limita-

---

9. Feuillet L, Dufour H, Pelletier, J. 2007. (See full reference in caption for figure 29.)

tions. It is a very illustrative example that shows us the extent to which the brain adapts to specific circumstances and demands. In this case, even with only 25 percent of its mass, the brain was capable of developing all the functions that are generally distributed and shared in a whole brain mass. In less extreme cases, it has also been observed that brain regions that were not originally intended to perform certain functions can take over the same functions when needed.

Recently, this plastic capacity of the brain has not only been conceived as an automatic attribute of the brain that appears in cases of need, but a vast and extensive line of research has been developed to design strategies that enhance neuroplasticity, and thus obtain therapeutic benefits, both in neurodegenerative diseases and in psychological disorders, pain, and other pathologies.

This strategy is more aligned with the aspects related to the biological complexity of our organism, as well as with the diseases that afflict it, which we already discussed in the first chapter. In the face of neurodegenerative diseases, for example, it seems absolutely unsuccessful (although still being attempted) to apply the classic model of drug development, looking for some specific targets related to the development of the disease and using drugs that modulate them. It's like trying to put out a fire in a twenty-story building using a fire extinguisher. The promotion of neuroplasticity, on the other hand, does not seek to attack specific targets, but rather to provide the brain with sufficient capacity to "manage" an illness and regain its power of adaptation. Instead of spending our energies trying to put out the fire with a fire extinguisher, we would call the fire department, evacuate everyone inside, secure the area, contain the flames wherever we could, and so on. However, sticking to the specific example of neurodegenerative diseases, no one should think that this one strategy would solve them. When the disease is already established, there are too many failures at too many levels in all systems: there are impairments in the speed of processing, in local responses and in the coordination between different systems, in the inhibitory controls of neuronal function, in the temporal representation of stimuli (rhythmic sequences, intervals), in the abstract representation of situations and scenarios, in working memory, selective attention, elementary predictions, motor and physiological control, in the direction of thought, and so on. Therefore, it is still unlikely that the induction of neuroplasticity would solve the inherent complexity in failures of this type. However, we insist that it is an innovative and valuable approach, which perhaps in the future will allow the development of strategies that do have the potential to be more effective in the treatment of these diseases.

It is also true that the induction of neuroplasticity, by itself, does not have to be therapeutic or produce benefits. There are two crucial aspects to keep in mind when we want to apply neuroplasticity to any disease. First, in what regions this plasticity is going to be expressed. Depending on the strategy used to increase brain plasticity, the regions that will end up benefitting from it may be different. For example, in transcranial magnetic stimulation, a technique that is currently on the rise and that promotes brain plasticity, the region of interest in which to intervene is selected very precisely, so that in addictions or depression it is useless to stimulate brain plasticity in the occipital cortex, let's say, where visual information is integrated. However, pharmacological techniques to induce neuroplasticity, which could include the use of psychedelics, do not have the ability to be so precise.

In the case of ibogaine, for example, it has been observed in animal studies that it increases neuroplasticity mainly in the nucleus accumbens (very involved in addictions and emotional processing), in the substantia nigra (crucial in Parkinson's disease), and in the prefrontal cortex (involved in addictions and also in a large number of cognitive tasks). But, again, when it comes to neuroplasticity, we cannot use the same logic that is used in traditional drugs, according to which we will obtain certain effects if we activate or deactivate a certain receptor. The simple induction of plasticity is not something inherently "positive" or desirable. In fact, it could happen that a greater plasticity in the nucleus accumbens produces greater facility in establishing an addictive habit. The only thing that allows us to know that this is not the case is clinical evidence, but there is no *baseline* that makes us think that the induction of plasticity in that region will be therapeutic. Greater plasticity can translate, broadly speaking and in general, into greater adaptation. And adaptation is neither good nor bad; it is a neutral concept. While it may have some benefits, adapting to certain circumstances may actually be counterproductive, the associated advantages or disadvantages being a mere matter of perspective. For example, if the brain receives a daily dose of heroin, it is adaptive to get used to it, but at the family level it may not be an adaptive pattern, due to the possible consequences on the family economy itself or on the ability to work and be productive.

Another crucial aspect to consider are the conditions in which we induce greater plasticity. This can be clearly seen when we look at plasticity in the context of physical rehabilitation, be it after an accident or some kind of trauma. If we induce plasticity in this context but do not exercise the affected body parts, recovery will be just as slow or even slower. However, if in the context of performing regular rehabilitation exercises we introduce an element that enhances plasticity, recovery will be much faster. This example, which can be intuitively understood, has taken many years to be recognized in the context of depression or other psychological disorders. Inducing plasticity in a person who suffers from depression and who does not leave the house or go to psychotherapy or any social activity, will surely have no effect. However, stimulating plasticity in a person with depression who is seeing a therapist on a weekly basis, who forces themselves to go swimming or attend some kind of workshop from time to time and even to take long walks in the morning, will likely have a powerful therapeutic effect. The latest findings on the use of antidepressants point in this direction, which suggest that these drugs should not be used as if they were an antibiotic acting on its own (without needing us to do our part), but should only be prescribed in the context of enhancing broader psychotherapeutic interventions. The same must be applied in the case of psychedelics, since, despite enhancing plasticity and inducing psychological experiences with a transformative potential, their efficacy can only be considered in the context of a previously established psychotherapy.

Neurological Evidence of Psychedelics' Therapeutic Effects

Before presenting the main evidence on the therapeutic effects of psychedelics obtained through neuroimaging techniques, we need to give another warning about the reliability of these techniques. Although they are very useful and have allowed great advances in the fields of therapeutics and research, their extensive and remarkable limitations are often not considered. Let me provide an example. In 2009, a rather surprising study was published[10] in which Craig Bennett, then a Ph.D. student, had put a salmon (dead, albeit fresh) in the MRI machine, initially to run some tests and make sure everything was working properly before performing the MRIs on the people participating in their study. To verify the entire process, he simulated the conditions and procedures of the study, so the salmon was presented with images of people interacting in social settings while being verbally asked to focus on what emotions those people were feeling. What was surprising was that the data, which were not corrected for multiple comparisons,[11] showed activations in the spinal cord and some brain regions of the dead salmon (see figure 30). This would be nothing more than an anecdote if all neuroimaging studies corrected for multiple comparisons, but the truth is that before the publication of the salmon study, about 40 percent of the published studies did not. After Bennett's publication, it is estimated that now only 10 percent of the studies do not correct their data for multiple comparisons, a percentage that is still very high given the risks involved in relation to the theories and hypotheses on which scientific work is based. One of the reasons why many researchers do not apply this correction is

---

10. Bennett CM, Wolford GL, Miller MB. 2009. The principled control of false positives in neuroimaging. Social Cognitive and Affective Neuroscience 4(4):417–422.

11. Multiple comparison correction is a basic procedure in statistics, practically obligatory in cases where many analyses are carried out and where there are many possibilities of finding false positives. "Correcting" basically means increasing the cutoff point from which some results are statistically significant, thus making it more difficult to reach that cutoff point and interpreting the results more conservatively.

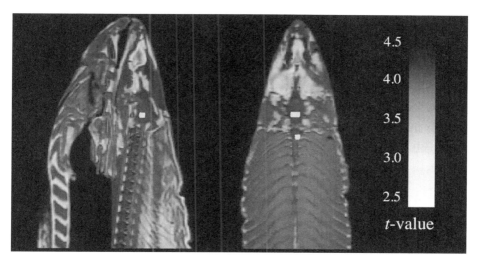

Figure 30. Brain activity reported by magnetic resonance imaging in a specimen of *Salmo salar* (salmon), while being shown images of individuals of the *Homo sapiens* species interacting. Original image adapted from the article cited in note 10 of this chapter: Bennett, Wolford, and Miller (2009). Reproduced with the authors' permission. (See also color plate 12.)

as simple as the fact that if they did, they might not get meaningful results. Unfortunately, it is common to prefer publishing something meaningful but dishonest over publishing nothing or publishing unremarkable or unimpressive results.

Beyond the correction or not of multiple comparisons, the use of neuroimaging techniques has also been criticized a lot because, although it allows us to "see" what happens to the brain while performing a task or under the influence of some psychedelic, lots of information is lost along the way. Much of what ends up being observed and interpreted as "activations" or "deactivations" is actually the result of complex interactions at the cellular level, which are by no means homogeneous and consistent. Trying to understand what's going on in the brain from an MRI is literally like trying to figure out what's going on at a party by looking at the lights coming out of your house windows. Despite this, we insist that they are also very useful techniques, especially due to the fact that they are not invasive, and that, when used and interpreted correctly, they can provide very valuable information.

In the case of psychedelics, enough neuroimaging studies have been performed to describe some general patterns of how they affect brain function. For example, through proton emission tomography (PET) or single-photon emission computed tomography (SPECT), mescaline, psilocybin, and ayahuasca induce fairly consistent activation patterns of the frontal cortex or the medial temporal lobe (structure located below the cortex and where the hippocampus is located, for example). Both techniques (PET and SPECT) consist of obtaining brain images through radioactive drugs that are injected intravenously. These drugs are called "tracers," basically because when they enter the systemic circulation and subsequently the brain, they allow us to "see" the blood flow that is distributed in each brain region. It is as if these drugs "illuminate" the flow of blood so that it shows up well in the brain images obtained. By observing blood flow, brain activation is also inferred, since those areas that are more active will require more oxygen and glucose, therefore demanding more irrigation, and an increase in blood flow will appear.

Other neuroimaging studies have also used functional magnetic resonance imaging (fMRI). This technique makes it possible to see brain activation patterns more directly and, furthermore, is less invasive, as it does not require the injection of radioactive drugs. Studies that have used fMRI report less consistent results, showing some divergence. For example, in a study[12] in which psilocybin was administered to healthy volunteers, reductions in connectivity were observed between the thalamus (main brain region related to processing and filtering sensory stimuli) and other brain regions, while in another study[13] in which

12. Carhart-Harris RL, Erritzoe D, Williams T, Stone JM, Reed LJ, Colasanti A, Tyacke RJ, Leech R, Malizia AL, Murphy K, et al. 2012. Neural correlates of the psychedelic state as determined by fMRI studies with psilocybin. Proceedings of the National Academy of Sciences of the United States of America 109(6):2138–2143.
13. Tagliazucchi E, Carhart-Harris R, Leech R, Nutt D, Chialvo DR. 2014. Enhanced repertoire of brain dynamical states during the psychedelic experience. Human Brain Mapping 35(11):5442–5456.

psilocybin was also used, greater functional connectivity was reported in different networks, such as the default mode network (DMN) or the executive control network. Currently, it is considered that psilocybin, especially, causes less "local" activation of different regions or neural networks, while increasing the connectivity between them.

Since the DMN has been mentioned, it is important to highlight that one of the key mechanisms believed to be related to the potential benefits of psychedelics is precisely the dissolution of the DMN. This neural network is particularly active in states associated with mind-wandering, and its activation decreases as we focus on specific tasks. Increased activity in this network has also been observed in individuals with various psychopathologies.

In most cases, arguments mentioning the DMN tend to be reductionist and exhibit several biases. The disruption of the DMN by psychedelics may occur because they induce a cognitively demanding experience where one confronts the "task" of one's subconscious, wrestling with the profound metaphysical and personal questions that typically emerge during such experiences. In other words, as something captivating all our attention occurs, the DMN is obviously going to be inactive, just as when we are cooking, fixing our bike, or jotting down tomorrow's tasks in our planner.

In fact, it is not even necessary to engage in any activity: the simple awareness of mind-wandering, as observed in meditation, reduces the resting functional connectivity of the DMN. Therefore, when contextualizing all these observations regarding changes in the DMN's configuration, the effects of psychedelics appear less like magic and more like a common correlate also present in numerous daily activities. In fact, the alterations observed in the DMN following psychedelic use bear resemblance to those reported after the administration of selective serotonin reuptake inhibitors (SSRIs).[14] This suggests that the changes might represent unspecific serotonergic effects. As the authors of a

---

14. Klaassens BL, van Gorsel HC, Khalili-Mahani N, et al. 2015. Single-dose serotonergic stimulation shows widespread effects on functional brain connectivity. NeuroImage 122:440–50.

recent review on the subject say: "Although the DMN is consistently implicated in psychedelic studies, it is unclear how central the DMN is to the therapeutic potential of classical psychedelic agents."[15]

Indeed, I would take a step further and question whether it is always necessary to act on this network and to always consider such disruption of the DMN as desirable. For certain individuals with very rigid mental patterns or high levels of neuroticism, a relaxation of activity related to a sustained hyperactivation of the DMN may be beneficial. However, for others facing different issues, such disruption may not be desirable.

Another pattern that has also been observed in the case of the most studied psychedelics, such as psilocybin, consists of a reduction in activity in regions associated with fear or anxiety, especially the amygdala (a structure closely related to emotional processing and especially fear or aversion). Although there are also divergences in this sense, because when psilocybin has been administered to healthy volunteers,[16] a lower reactivity of the amygdala to aversive stimuli was observed one week after administration, an effect that is maintained up to one month after administration. However, when psilocybin has been administered to patients with depression,[17] a greater reactivity of the amygdala was registered twenty-four hours after taking it, something that a priori would not be desirable in this population. This pattern of deactivation of the amygdala (especially in a healthy population) is not found in substances such as salvinorin-A, which precisely activates many subcortical regions, including the amygdala. Despite inducing generalized decreases in activity in cortical areas and

15. Gattuso JJ, Perkins D, Ruffell S, et al. 2023. Default mode network modulation by psychedelics: a systematic review. International Journal of Neuropsychopharmacology 26(3):155–188.
16. Barrett FS, Doss MK, Sepeda ND, Pekar JJ, Griffiths RR. 2020. Emotions and brain function are altered up to one month after a single high dose of psilocybin. Scientific Reports 10(1):2214.
17. Roseman L, Demetriou L, Wall MB, Nutt DJ, Carhart-Harris RL. 2018. Increased amygdala responses to emotional faces after psilocybin for treatment-resistant depression. Neuropharmacology 142:263–269.

activating subcortical regions, such as the amygdala, it has been suggested that salvinorin-A would also have an antidepressant effect, so it is advisable, once again, not to be guided solely and myopically by the findings in neuroimaging studies.

In the case of ayahuasca, in a study[18] where it was administered to healthy volunteers, reductions in functional connectivity of the DMN were observed. These results were interpreted as a positive effect of ayahuasca, as DMN hyperactivation is associated with multiple psychopathologies, from depression to schizophrenia. In fact, the DMN is the neural network that is most active when we are not doing anything, when we are unable to concentrate or not focusing our attention on any particular point or activity. In this sense, activities such as meditation or reading are associated with reductions in DMN activity. However, we must interpret these results with caution, since it is not so clear that a decrease in functional connectivity in the DMN is actually desirable.

Functional connectivity is a parameter that reports the level of connection and communication between the different brain regions that make up a neural network. When this functional connectivity is high, it is assumed that there is good communication between these regions and that there is poor communication when the functional connectivity is low. Although the term *networks* is used to understand how the brain works, it should be noted that these networks do not actually exist; they are just patterns of communication between different regions of the brain. Therefore, when we speak of low functional connectivity, it is not that any network is deactivated; it is just that the regions that encompass it stop working as they usually do, and for this reason we can no longer speak of a "network," since these regions stop receiving or sending nerve impulses to other regions. This should inform the degree of abstraction and artificiality of the terms used in the field of

18. Palhano-Fontes F, Andrade KC, Tofoli LF, Santos AC, Crippa JAS, Hallak JEC, Ribeiro S, de Araujo DB. 2015. The psychedelic state induced by ayahuasca modulates the activity and connectivity of the default mode network. PLoS One 10(2):e0118143.

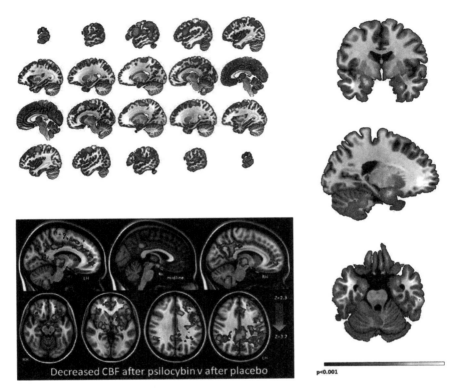

Figure 31. Variations in cerebral blood flow after administration of salvinorin-A (*top* and *right*) and psilocybin (*bottom*). In the case of salvinorin-A, extensive decreases in blood flow were reported in the cortex of all cerebral lobes (frontal, temporal, medial, and occipital) and increases in flow in subcortical regions, mainly the amygdala, hippocampus, and cerebellum. Psilocybin, by contrast, only showed more discreet decreases in blood flow in some regions of the cortex and in subcortical regions, such as the thalamus. No flux increase was observed in this case.

The images on the effects of salvinorin-A are partially published in the article: Ona G, Sampedro F, Romero S, Valle M, Camacho V, Migliorelli C, Mañanas MÁ, Antonijoan RM, Puntes M, Coimbra J, et al. 2022. The kappa-opioid receptor and the sleep of reason: cortico-subcortical imbalance following salvinorin-A. The International Journal of Neuropsychopharmacology 25(1):54–63. The psilocybin image originally appeared in the article: Carhart-Harris RL, Erritzoe D, Williams T, Stone JM, Reed LJ, Colasanti A, Tyacke RJ, Leech R, Malizia AL, Murphy K, et al. 2012. Neural correlates of the psychedelic state as determined by fMRI studies with psilocybin. Proceedings of the National Academy of Sciences of the United States of America 109(6): 2138–2143. All images reproduced with the authors' permission. (See also color plate 13.)

neuroimaging. Moreover, if we speak in these terms and assume that there is a deactivation of the DMN when ayahuasca is taken, we cannot say this is a desirable result. In fact, it has been observed that people who show poor functional connectivity of the DMN also have difficulties in deactivating this network and giving way to other networks. When they go from being unfocused to focusing on a task that requires concentration, the DMN is not completely deactivated and some of its regions remain very active, contrary to people who do show greater functional connectivity in the DMN. It is as if the brain needed all its networks to work very well (have high functional connectivity) so that the transition from one network to another is also very clear and efficient. Therefore, the fact that ayahuasca "deactivates" the DMN may be good news in a context of psychopathology and as a temporary intervention to facilitate some psychotherapeutic processes, but in the medium or long term, we may be more interested in having a highly functional DMN, so that its deactivation is also functional. It is these effects, in the medium or long term, that are still unknown.

In the case of LSD, in a study[19] in which it was administered to healthy volunteers, a reduction in the functional connectivity of the DMN was also observed. In addition, this study was widely publicized in the media, since a correlation was also found between the reduction in functional connectivity in the DMN and the subjective experience of "ego dissolution."[20] Had the neural correlate of the foundations of the mystical experience, the cerebral basis of the death experience that so many people have tirelessly sought for centuries, finally been found? Unfortunately, not everything was so pretty (as is often the case in

---

19. Carhart-Harris RL, Muthukumaraswamy S, Roseman L, Kaelen M, Droog W, Murphy K, Tagliazucchi E, Schenberg EE, Nest T, Orban C, et al. 2016. Neural correlates of the LSD experience revealed by multimodal neuroimaging. Proceedings of the National Academy of Sciences of the United States of America 113(17):4853–4858.
20. The experience of "ego dissolution" occurs when there is a marked loss of the sense of individual identity, giving way to a connection or identification with large groups, society, and all forms of life.

science). The study was replicated by Swiss researchers[21] and no such association was found. In fact, the same researchers from the first study later acknowledged that their results were highly questionable, since the exact same phenomenon had been observed when using selective serotonin reuptake inhibitors (SSRIs, the most commonly used antidepressants), which, of course, do not induce any experience of "ego dissolution," although they generate the same pattern from the standpoint of neuroimaging. This suggests that the effects observed when using LSD are not specific to this substance, and that they would be, at best, related to serotonin or other phenomena that occur with both LSD and SSRIs. In conclusion, the characterization of the functionality of neural networks is only a model that tries to explain, in an extremely simple way, very complex phenomena and experiences, which is why divergent, contradictory, or directly erroneous results are often found. It is possible that in the future, using other techniques that enrich the information obtained, the effects of psychedelics on the brain and the basis for their therapeutic potential might be better explained.

Finally, apart from neural network analyses, anatomical differences in the brain have also been found, possibly caused by the continued use of some psychedelics. For example, in a study carried out at the Hospital de la Santa Creu i Sant Pau in Barcelona, where "veteran" ayahuasca consumers were recruited (the criterion was established as having consumed ayahuasca at least fifty times), the subjects showed greater cortical thickness in a region called the anterior cingulate cortex, compared to nonconsumers of ayahuasca. In fact, the more times they had consumed ayahuasca, the greater this difference. When we talk about "thickness," we really talk about neuronal bodies, gray matter. Having greater cortical thickness in this area, in theory, is something positive, since the presence of mood disorders has traditionally been associated with less cortical thickness in this specific area, although again we need to enact caution in interpreting these results, since it is not possible to completely estab-

---

21. Mueller F, Dolder PC, Schmidt A, Liechti ME, Borgwardt S. 2018. Altered network hub connectivity after acute LSD administration. Neuroimaging Clinics of North America 18:694–701.

lish causality between the consumption of ayahuasca and an increase in cortical thickness. It is possible that these people already had a greater cortical thickness before the start of consumption, something that will never be verifiable. In any case, this was the first evidence of plasticity and brain anatomical changes induced by ayahuasca.

Hormonal Effects

Most psychedelics also cause a release of some hormones and peptides,[22] mainly because the hypothalamus (the main production center of these substances) has a high density of 5-HT2A receptors. Especially MDMA and LSD have been associated with increases in the levels of oxytocin, a hormone highly involved in social ties, love, and affection. The administration of pure oxytocin when undergoing psychotherapeutic treatment has also been associated with substantial improvements, so it seems especially clear that the therapeutic use of psychedelics also induces the release of this hormone.

Ayahuasca and psilocybin also increase cortisol levels. This is relevant in the case of its use in people with depression, since it is precisely the main indication for which they are being studied. In fact, in a recent study,[23] it was observed that people with depression indeed had significantly lower cortisol levels than the control group, which did not have depression. After the administration of a single dose of ayahuasca, cortisol levels increased to where there were no differences with respect to the control group and remained there for at least forty-eight hours. In conclusion, the neuroendocrine effects of psychedelics are highly relevant in terms of their therapeutic use, and especially in patients with depression.

---

22. Peptides are small amino acids involved in a large number of functions. Examples of peptides are oxytocin and insulin.
23. Osório FdL, Sanches RF, Macedo LR, Santos RG, Maia de Oliveira JP, Wichert-Ana L, Araujo DB, Riba J, Crippa JAS, Hallak JEC. 2015. Antidepressant effects of a single dose of ayahuasca in patients with recurrent depression: a preliminary report. British Journal of Psychiatry 37(1):13–20.

Psychological Effects

Although a later section has been reserved exclusively to discuss the psychoactive effects of psychedelic drugs, we need to dedicate a few lines to mentioning them in this section, since they are an important part of their therapeutic effects. It should be remembered, in fact, that few times in the history of psychology and psychiatry have we come across pharmacological treatments that induce therapeutic effects through the subjective experiences they immediately facilitate, with the exception of Moreau de Tours and his experiments with hashish and belladonna, or later Humphry Davy (1778–1829; British chemist) with nitrous oxide, among a few examples. The design of therapeutic programs with specific administrations of psychedelic drugs, in which patients are accompanied by their therapists on a transformative journey, is a paradigm shift in psychotherapeutic practice.

First of all, the psychological effects that these drugs induce allow subjects to live deeply significant and meaningful personal experiences, to access states of clear and increased introspection, and to strengthen the relationship with their therapists. "Peak experiences," as A. Maslow called them, or mystical experiences, have great potential for psychological advancement and enrichment and, in fact, the appearance and quality of these experiences have been correlated with their therapeutic benefits, the latter being more marked the more intense and complete the experiences were. It is also common to experience feelings and sensations of fascination or stupefaction, either when facing some aesthetically beautiful stimulus, such as a flower or a painting, or facing existence itself. The ability to feel this fascination, as well as its effects on our psyche, have also often been included among the psychological benefits of psychedelics.

Some variables of psychological processing also tend to be altered after experiences with psychedelics. This has been reflected in studies with ayahuasca, where an increase in "decentering" was observed, that is, in the ability to detach and dissociate oneself from one's own sufferings, thus reducing their impact. Personality can also be susceptible to some changes after intense experiences with psychedelics. In particular, increases in some personality traits such as "openness to experience" or "optimism" have been reported.

It is essential to highlight an implicit error that has been systematically made in many studies on psychedelics. It has been assumed that these psychological effects, these peak experiences characterized by the appreciation of life's profound beauty and enormous transformative potential, will be replicated in all subjects. Most researchers in the field—we can now say this clearly—are working on this because they have had very positive experiences with psychedelics in the past and deduce that these experiences could be beneficial for people with mental disorders. However, this need not be the case. Carrying a mental health diagnosis for years represents a very complex and challenging reality, one that I am sure no one "on the other side," attending to these individuals, can imagine. I have often seen people with depression or other disorders receive high doses of *Psilocybe* mushrooms or ayahuasca and not experience anything close to the numinous—quite the opposite. And in a way, it is understandable. If your entire reality is in a dark pit where nothing makes sense, you feel no energy or motivation to engage in activities, and when you do, you derive no pleasure from them, perhaps you are not in a moment that is conducive to experiencing one of the highest self-realization experiences of the human psyche. Assuming that a certain type of experience will be induced in any person simply by administering a certain molecule at a certain dose is more characteristic of a biomedical model that applies naive and simplistic logic to much more complex realities. We should bear this in mind when discussing the experiences these substances often elicit.

MICRODOSING PSYCHEDELICS AS AN EMERGING TREND

Part of the therapeutic potential of psychedelics that is being explored is the use of very small doses (microdoses) more or less continuously. Microdoses, despite not inducing relevant psychological effects, have some benefits that have aroused the interest of both scientists

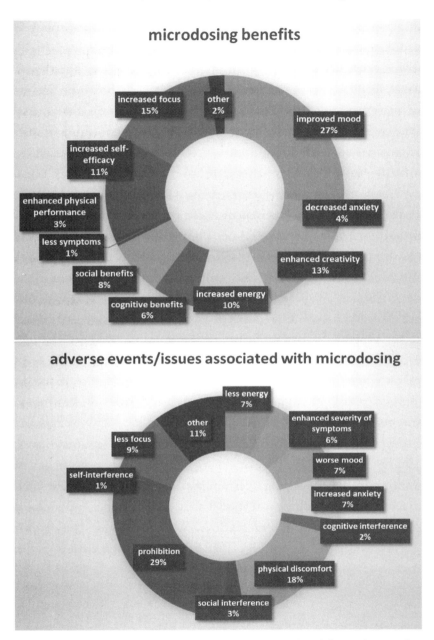

Figure 32. The image has been adapted and translated from the article: Anderson T, Petranker R, Christopher A, Rosenbaum D, Weissman C, Dinh-Williams L-A, Hui K, Hapke E. 2019. Psychedelic microdosing benefits and challenges: an empirical codebook. Harm Reduction Journal 16:43. (See also color plate 14.)

and the general population, being a practice in clear expansion.

Psilocybin mushrooms or LSD are generally used to prepare micro-doses, although ibogaine or ayahuasca are also used, among other psychedelics. The main applications of microdoses are for the increase of cognitive performance, for example, in employees in very demanding fields, such as computing, design, or scientific research itself; in the empowerment of creativity in artists or intellectuals; in increased mood; and in the treatment of some physical or psychological symptoms, dependencies, and the like. It has also been reported in some case studies that microdoses of ibogaine could be useful in treating certain symptoms of Parkinson's disease. This line of research has not yet produced results that can point in one direction or another, although studies are already being carried out with LSD in the geriatric population for the possible treatment of other neurodegenerative diseases.

The first systematic review[24] that analyzed the results of all published studies on the phenomenon of microdosing psychedelics collected data from some three thousand users. Improved mood and increased creativity and energy were often cited among the benefits of this practice. On the other hand, the presence of side effects, such as insomnia, feelings of strangeness or discomfort, and headache, were also reported. This suggests that even low doses that are not psychoactive may not have a safety profile that is entirely favorable.

Despite the fact that some studies have confirmed the induction of analgesia using microdoses of LSD, as well as the release of neurotrophic factors after its use, there are still serious doubts about the amount of placebo effect there could be in the supposed benefits of microdoses. Considering that many, if not most, microdosing users have also consumed regular doses of the same psychedelics and that a regular dose of these induces highly relevant and remarkable psychological experiences, mere contact with the same substance could induce benefits by suggestion or, at least, a good predisposition.

---

24. Ona G, Bouso JC. 2020. Potential safety, benefits, and influence of the placebo effect in microdosing psychedelic drugs: a systematic review. Neuroscience and Biobehavioral Reviews 119:194–203.

ADVERSE EFFECTS IN THE THERAPEUTIC
USE OF PSYCHEDELICS

In my early university years, I was somewhat of a psychedelics enthusiast. Though I didn't consume them regularly or frequent places where they were widely used, such as raves, electronic music venues, or festivals (I quickly discovered how pleasant it is to stay home on a Saturday night with your cat), I was always intellectually intrigued by them. Consequently, I immersed myself in both the formal and informal literature on the subject and became well-versed in the optimal conditions for safe use, known as "set and setting." As a result, many students would seek my advice before trying LSD or mushrooms for the first time. This often led me, in addition to having long conversations with the students before and after their experiences (what would today be conceptualized as preparation and integration, though I didn't use these terms at the time), to also be present during their use and create a comfortable and serene setting with blankets, dim lighting, incense, precious stones, art books, evocative music, nature documentaries, acrylic paints and canvases, and so forth. All with the goal of providing a special aesthetic experience and facilitating peak experiences. Over two or three years, I accompanied more than one hundred people, and the majority of the experiences were memorable. I remember those as some of the best years of my life because I had the privilege of witnessing very significant moments in many people's lives. However, I vividly remember the first two people I advised. They were two girls. Both had a positive and very special experience during the session. We had it at one of their houses by the beach during the off-season, so there was no one else around and we were able to enjoy a wonderful day. However, while one of them continued to feel notably positive effects in the days and weeks after the experience, the other entered a hell from which it took her over a year and many hours of therapy to recover. She would often experience psychedelic effects, especially when consuming cannabis, leading her into very unpleasant mental loops that ended in anxiety and panic attacks. The only advice I could offer her at the time was to stay away from any substances and to see a psychologist. She did and, as I mentioned, it took her just over a year to recover. This was the first warning (among others that I would encounter) about the risks of psychedelics. I can't help but feel a certain irritation, therefore, when certain individuals assert emphatically that these substances are very safe and will probably have no negative consequences. As we will see, there is still much to learn.

> Pharmacology is combined with toxicology when studying physiological responses to any drug that could be considered adverse, or what are known as side effects.

The use of these drugs makes it necessary to know in detail the potential risks and the mechanisms by which toxicity is induced in the body. The truth is that all medicines, once authorized for marketing, enter what is called phase IV, where they are continuously monitored and evaluated, compiling side effects that doctors or patients have reported after using or being exposed to the medicines in question. This is known as pharmacovigilance. In the event that serious side effects are reported over the years or if they do not compensate for the benefits obtained by the medication (hair loss due to an interruption of cell proliferation mechanisms may be acceptable in the event of suffering a potentially fatal cancer, but it would not be so in the case of suffering from osteoarthritis, for example), the competent agencies may decide to withdraw the authorization for the marketing of a given drug and thus remove it from the market. That's what happened to rimonabant (an antagonist of cannabinoid receptors), Myolastan, and many others.

Toxicity

Most psychedelic drugs have little physiological toxicity. However, it is crucial to distinguish between toxicity and pharmacological effects. The absence of physiological toxicity does not preclude the potential for significant adverse events, which fall under the domain of pharmacology.

Therefore, while psychedelic drugs may exhibit minimal physiological toxicity, it is important to consider their profound pharmacological impacts, which can lead to serious psychological or neurological effects. In fact, the effects of psychedelic drugs on a psychological level are unpredictable, and there have been lots of accidents (falls, crashes, blows . . .) reported in relation to the consumption of psychedelics. Regarding its physiological toxicity, cases have been reported in which massive doses of LSD were accidentally taken without serious adverse reactions (without going any further, the previously mentioned case in which a woman mistook her LSD for cocaine, snorting a dose 550 times higher than a normal dose of LSD, without serious consequences). Other extremely physiologically safe psychedelics are psilocybin and DMT.

However, some psychedelics do have associated toxicity. For example, high doses of mescaline have been associated with serious adverse effects, mainly cardiovascular, and there are even some documented deaths caused by mescaline. Another uncommon adverse reaction, but one to be taken into account, is rhabdomyolysis. This occurs when skeletal muscle is damaged and muscle fibers are released into the systemic circulation, causing damage to a large number of tissues or organs, especially the kidneys. It is a serious condition that can lead to kidney failure, encephalopathy, and, if left untreated, possible death. Generally, it is cocaine, heroin, or statins (medicines for cholesterol control) that most often cause rhabdomyolysis. However, there are documented cases in which it has occurred after the consumption of LSD and psilocybin mushrooms. Although it is a rare phenomenon, it should be taken into consideration in people with impaired kidney function or with a medical problem that inhibits the metabolism of these substances.

MDMA, or rather its metabolism, as we saw in previous sections, also has some toxic effects on various organs and systems. First, liver toxicity has been described and, in fact, many intoxications with high doses of MDMA cause jaundice, that is, a yellowish skin tone, with some hemorrhage or increased liver enzymes. Second, there appears to be cardiovascular toxicity as well, primarily related to the ability of MDMA to induce norepinephrine release. This is harmful to the cardiovascular system, because it increases blood pressure and heart rate, with the subsequent risk of ruptured vessels, hemorrhages, tachycardia, and other phenomena that overload cardiac function. Finally, neurotoxicity associated with the consumption of MDMA has also been reported. This would be associated not with the substance itself, but with the contexts in which it is usually used. In clubs or raves, where the body is subjected to intense physical activity, and due to the alteration in the regulation of body temperature caused by MDMA, generally users sweat a lot and lose large amounts of sodium. As a result, they often drink large amounts of water, so sodium concentrations are further diluted, leading to a medical condition called hyponatremia, where sodium levels are extremely low. In conditions of hyponatremia, the water contained in the blood passes into the tissues, including the brain, causing the appearance of seizures and compression of the brainstem and cerebellum, running the risk of having basic functions regulated from these areas, such as breathing or heart rate, interrupted. Of course, it is convenient to assess at what dose levels and in what contexts these effects can occur, since, in the clinical trials carried out to date, with controlled doses and conditions, no serious adverse effects have yet been reported.

Ibogaine is another psychedelic substance that poses some considerable risks on a physiological level. It seems that at very low doses (microdoses, no more than 20 or 30 mg) it has stimulant effects. However, there are discrepancies on that regard. When Dybowski and Landrin, two French explorers, in the nineteenth century asked the Indigenous groups of the Congo about the *Tabernanthe iboga* plant's effects, they replied that "the action of iboga was identical to that of alcohol, but without disturbing thought processes." From that statement, the researchers understood that the plant was used as a stimulant. However, these Indigenous groups might have been more inclined to draw a comparison between the iboga plant and the Kola nut (*Cola nitida*) if their intention was to describe its stimulant effects, as they were using both plants often. Based on our current knowledge, a dose of 20 mg of ibogaine does not produce stimulating effects and does not appear to significantly affect cognitive performance in a controlled clinical setting.[25] Thus, this contemporary finding seem to align more closely with the comparison made by the carriers of iboga's traditional knowledge, who likened its effects to those of alcohol. Once the ibogaine dose is increased to 100 or 200 mg, feelings of relaxation and well-being are induced, without alterations in the electrocardiogram (ECG). As doses approach 400–500 mg or more, psychoactive effects appear and an ECG parameter called the QT interval lengthens (see figure 33). This interval is measured in milliseconds, and when it exceeds 500 or 550 ms is

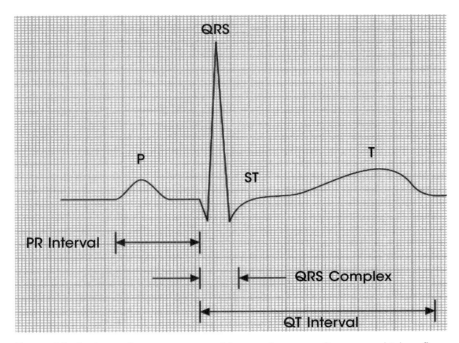

Figure 33. Section of waves reported by an electrocardiogram, which reflect the electrical activity of the heart. These waves always follow the same order: first comes the P wave, followed by Q (the subtle downward peak before the big upward peak), the R wave (the highest peak), the S (the small indentation after R), and finally the T wave. The interval between the Q and T waves is called the QT interval. This is measured in milliseconds (ms), and normal values are generally between 400 and 450 ms.

25. Forsyth, B, Machado L, Jowett T, Jakobi H, Garbe K, Winter H, Glue P. 2016. Effects of low dose ibogaine on subjective mood state and psychological performance. Journal of Ethnopharmacology 189:10–13.

when certain problems can appear, such as malignant arrhythmias and, in the worst cases, death. This is why the cardiotoxicity of ibogaine is often talked about. There have been a few dozen deaths associated with the use of ibogaine, generally due to mixing it with other substances, the presence of other medical problems, or taking doses that are too high, although it has also occurred in people with no previous history of other diseases or usage of other drugs. The safety profile of ibogaine has still hardly been studied, and the maximum tolerated dose (MTD) and the minimum effective dose (MED), parameters widely used in pharmacology and that guide the dosage of each medication, remain unknown. Other problems that ibogaine can cause, especially at high doses, are vomiting and nausea, seizures, loss of consciousness, ataxia, or muscle rigidity, among others.

Scopolamine and atropine are perhaps the perfect example that the difference between a remedy and a poison lies in the dose. If adequate amounts of these substances are used, they are highly effective and useful, but at inadequate doses they produce often lethal effects. Scopolamine, even at therapeutic doses, can cause fatigue, amnesia, or vertigo. In addition, it increases the pressure of the eyeball, therefore it should not be used in people suffering from glaucoma. High doses induce seizures, vivid hallucinations, generalized excitement, irritability, or cognitive alterations, among other effects. Continued use generates dependence and its interruption, a withdrawal syndrome characterized by nausea, dizziness, vomiting, bradycardia, and hypotension.

The new tryptamines include some substances that are particularly toxic, although the safety profile of a large number of them is still unknown. For example, 5-MeO-DiPT causes cognitive deficits in animals, such as impairments in learning and memory processes. Its use has also been associated with rhabdomyolysis and kidney failure in humans. Another substance, "Bromo-DragonFLY," a psychedelic phenethylamine, has also been associated with the death of young people who consumed it at unknown doses. It should be emphasized that the risks of these new substances are often unknown, which is why their consumption among the young population seems especially worrying, especially since they do not always use these substances in the best contexts or in doses that are theoretically safe.

Studying the Safety of Psychedelics

Despite a growing number of clinical studies, the safety profile of many psychedelics is still unclear. This is due to the fact that adverse reactions can vary considerably between the healthy population and the clinical population, since generally, in published studies, small samples have been used and the adverse reactions that occurred during studies have not always been systematically collected using standardized tools.

The matter of the samples used is a highly worrying aspect, since the patients who have participated in clinical studies constitute an incredibly scarce profile. A high percentage of these (between 50 percent and 75 percent) had previous experience with psychedelics. The authors tend to select patients with previous experience with these drugs and who, furthermore, have not developed problems derived from their use in the past. Thus, it is ensured that the person will react well to the psychedelic experience and will not suffer from bad trips or, worse still, psychotic or bipolar outbreaks. It is a way to guarantee their safety and it is absolutely understandable. However, this is detrimental to the external validity of the results obtained, that is, the extrapolation of the results to other populations. In other words: there can be no guarantee that other patients, other than those who participated in the study, will have the same benefits or harms.

The percentages, in clinical studies, of people with previous experience in the use of psychedelics (50–75 percent) seem high at first glance, but they seem even higher if we remember that the percentage of the general population that has ever consumed psychedelic drugs in their life is 1–2 percent, both in Europe and in the United States. After all, the effects of psychedelic drugs are popularly associated with madness and trips that are somewhat strange and eccentric, and they are not exactly the most popular drugs; far from it. It is that population in which only 1 percent is interested in psychedelic drugs that is expected to end up benefitting from their properties, so it is absurd to study them in populations belonging to that 1 percent rather than to the greater 99 percent. For the top 1 percent, the safety and efficacy profile of psychedelic drugs may be optimal, but by the time these substances are marketed, it may not be so optimal, and some patients will develop psychotic, bipolar, dissociative, or other disorders, so studies capable of describing the possible adverse effects of psychedelics should continue to be carried out.

Taking into account this possible underestimation of the adverse reactions of psychedelics, current studies have described a pattern of possible adverse reactions characterized by short-term and temporary manifestations, such as headache or anxiety. In addition, states of concern, confusion, or fear before taking these drugs have been associated with a greater probability of suffering adverse reactions. Conversely, people with high scores on "openness to experience" show fewer adverse reactions, indicating that intrapsychic factors actually play an important role in the occurrence of psychological adverse reactions.

In the case of psilocybin, for example,[26] in a recent study comparing psilocybin with escitalopram (an SSRI) in patients with depression, both substances induced more or less the same number of adverse reactions, with headache and nausea being the most common in the psilocybin group. In the ceremonial use of ayahuasca outside of clinical contexts, a study[27] reported an incidence of serious adverse reactions of 17.5 percent, consisting of physical aggression (from people who were having a difficult experience with their caregivers), loss of consciousness with and without seizures, or panic attacks. Among the most common nonserious adverse reactions, in the case of ayahuasca, are gastrointestinal symptoms, such as nausea or vomiting, although these are usually perceived as part of the experience, a "purge" necessary to

26. Carhart-Harris R, Giribaldi B, Watts R, Baker-Jones M, Murphy-Beiner A, Murphy R, Martell J, Blemings A, Erritzoe D, Nutt DJ. 2021. Trial of psilocybin versus escitalopram for depression. The New England Journal of Medicine 384(15):1402–1411.
27. Gómez-Sousa M, Jiménez-Garrido DF, Ona G, Dos Santos RG, Hallak J, Alcázar-Córcoles MÁ, Bouso JC. 2021. Acute psychological adverse reactions in first-time ritual ayahuasca users: a prospective case series. Journal of Clinical Psychopharmacology 41(2):163–171.

undertake deeper journeys. In the ceremonial use of psychedelics, such as ayahuasca, peyote, and others, the conditions are more conducive to containment and greater security, since there are often very experienced people who take care of the participants and can intervene quickly in any eventuality. Thus, ceremonial use would be preferable, in terms of safety, to recreational use, where there is less control and structure.

Health Risks When Using Psychedelic Drugs Therapeutically

It should be noted that the use of high doses of psychedelics can lead to vascular problems. Although the vast majority of psychedelics increase blood pressure and heart rate, these elevations are not clinically relevant at low or regular doses. However, the use of high doses could lead to problems, since the 5-HT2A receptor is associated with muscle contraction, thrombus (blood clot) formation, and coronary artery spasm; in short, effects derived mainly from vasoconstriction. This vasoconstriction would be responsible, for example, for psilocybin causing headaches, the severity of which is also dose dependent (the higher the dose, the greater the incidence, duration, and severity of the headache).

Another possible adverse reaction in the clinical or therapeutic use of psychedelics are "bad trips." This is how they are popularly referred to, although they are basically states of high anxiety, panic attacks, depersonalization, and so on. The intensity of the experience can often be overwhelming, especially with the use of moderate to high doses of psilocybin, LSD, or ayahuasca. The confrontation of certain experiences, relationships, or painful situations under the influence of psychedelic drugs is in fact something very challenging, since emotions are experienced in a more intense way, and it is also not possible to "flee" or "escape" from emerging psychological content, because distraction, or fixing the attention on other stimuli, is generally very complicated. In fact, in the psychotherapeutic approaches that deal with the design and development of models for psychedelic psychotherapy, it is assumed that it is much more advisable to surrender to the process and face these challenging or painful situations with an attitude of curiosity instead of trying to fight against them or avoid them. The problem has always been where to draw the line that separates "normal" anxiety symptoms, inherent in the confrontation of conflicting psychological material, from pathological anxiety symptoms that can cause major problems, or even make the person consider abandoning the psychotherapeutic process. This question is currently open and requires a calm and shared analysis with the maximum number of professionals possible, so that people who are going to undergo psychedelic-assisted psychotherapy can find themselves in a safe place at all times.

Finally, the most serious adverse reactions that can occur during the course of psychedelic drug use are exacerbation of psychotic and bipolar disorders, as well as hallucinogen persistent perception disorder (HPPD). In the case of psychotic and bipolar disorders, it seems that both psychedelic drugs and others (cocaine, amphetamines, or cannabis) could act as precipitators. That is, people with these vulnerabilities would be especially sensitive to developing these disorders after consumption. However, the diagnostic category that encompasses psychotic and bipolar disorders is very heterogeneous, and like all other psychiatric labels, it moves on a continuum where the presence of symptoms and traits is more or less accentuated, with people in the population with certain traits who in the near future will develop a disorder as such, as well as people who, with the same traits, will never develop one. The chances that one develops or not tend to increase, in theory, with exposure to risk factors: job insecurity, poverty, poor or unhealthy family ties, drug use, and so on.

It is considered that before the full development of a psychotic or bipolar disorder, that is, before the person's behavior is so manifestly aberrant, dangerous, or dysfunctional as to be seen by mental health professionals and receive a diagnosis, there is a previous phase where some symptoms appear, indicating the possible future development of the disorder. This phase is usually called the prodromal phase and intense work has been done to detect people in this phase. One of the most widely used paradigms in this regard is that of "high risk," through which, using different tools (clinical, psychometric, or genetic), the general population is screened in search of these people, in order to act preventively and avoid acute outbreaks that could easily end up threatening the physical or psychological integrity of the person who suffers it and the people around them. The problem is that, fortunately, not everyone who is in the prodromal phase ends up developing the disorder. As the psychology professor Inés Tomás used to say, it takes a lot to go crazy. That is why, if by means of these screenings we intervene with people who would not ultimately develop a disorder, there is a risk of overmedication, thus potentially causing high levels of iatrogenesis.

What the previous paragraph aims to say is that we do not know who will develop a psychotic or bipolar disorder in the future, although we are trying. Therefore, when a person is exposed to the use of psychedelics, there may be a small chance that this will happen. Generally, after the age of twenty to thirty, it is difficult for these disorders to develop, since they tend to appear at an early age, although there are always exceptions. Nor do they appear overnight. The person can spend a long time going through ayahuasca ceremonies, underground therapists who clandestinely administer psychedelics, or polysubstance use at raves before developing the disorder. But surely everything will increase the chances, so, again, as in the case of bad trips, it is necessary to develop the most effective preventive strategies possible, for example, following the evolution of patients for years to detect those individuals with higher risk, or fine-tuning the process of selection and admission of patients, so as not to accept those who also present certain traits that predispose them to the development of these disorders.

I can say that I have also contributed my part to this effort, as I developed a psychometric test[28] that measures the risk of developing psychotic and bipolar disorders, specifically designed to complement screening techniques in experimental or informal contexts where psy-

28. Ona, G. 2020. Elaboración y validación de un cuestionario para la detección del riesgo de reacciones adversas graves por empleo de drogas psicodélicas en terapia [Development and validation of a questionnaire to detect the risk of serious adverse reactions due to use of psychedelic drugs in therapy]. International Journal of Psychology and Psychological Therapy 20(2):211–22. Spanish.

chedelic substances are to be administered. To this day, we continue to rely on clinical judgment as the main tool for determining the risk or presence of psychotic or bipolar symptoms, as we do not have reliable biomarkers in this regard. Therefore, this test, which I developed using Samejima's Graded Response Model from Item Response Theory (IRT), offers a more objective measure than clinical judgment. Developing it through IRT was a real headache for me because it is mathematically very complex, but now it is a blessing. One of the advantages that IRT offers is that instruments can be developed that are not sensitive to the characteristics of the sample. Thus, the problem that most tests have regarding the variable reliability depending on the type of sample to which they are administered in this case disappears. The test always works in the same way and with the same precision (which is very high). It might seem like I'm selling a wonderful product for which you'll get a wonderful discount if you enter a code found at the end of the book in my online store, but none of that is so. Since I published the test, I have been providing it for free, as well as advising *pro bono* on its use and correction.

Let me add one final note of discord on this matter, as I am in favor of presenting other viewpoints even if they disagree with me or my work. Some researchers are suggesting that psychotic disorders may not be as related to psychedelics as previously thought. Perhaps in the future, these substances could be administered to individuals with such diagnoses. For instance, the brilliant Haley Maria Dourron is working on this. She conducted an intriguing survey among individuals diagnosed with psychotic disorders who reported that the substance producing effects most similar to their acute episodes was cannabis, not psychedelics. This and other evidence suggest that perhaps we have prevented people with psychotic disorders from being exposed to psychedelics out of sheer ignorance, assuming (without data) that this could be dangerous. This may change in the future.

As for HPPD, this is a category that has been included in different versions of the Diagnostic and Statistical Manual of Mental Disorders (DSM). It replaced another concept, "flashbacks," used since the 1960s, and which referred to the sudden appearance of symptoms identical to those caused by the ingestion of psychedelics (visual and auditory distortions, for example) long after having used them. However, recent studies have concluded that its staying power is really anecdotal and that this diagnostic category should be seriously questioned due to the fact that it is not possible to determine, based on the scientific research that has been carried out, that this phenomenon is actually possible after the use of psychedelics. The most plausible hypothesis at this time is that the cases in which HPPD has been reported are people with a special vulnerability, not related to psychotic or bipolar disorders, who, due to still unknown reasons, experience the effects of the substance at a later point, although, of course, these effects are no longer precipitated by the substance that was previously consumed.

PSYCHOACTIVE EFFECTS OF PSYCHEDELICS

The psychoactive effects produced by psychedelic drugs are a central feature within their pharmacodynamic evaluation. The reason why these effects occur is not known with great certainty, although the most accepted hypotheses point to a disruption of the activity of the thalamus, mediated by 5-HT2A receptors, which generally leads to a sensory overload of the cortex, producing the very common effects such as changes in emotional responses, perceptual and thought alterations, changes in visual imagery, or even modifications in one's own self-image or self-awareness.

Although we must emphasize once again the uniqueness of each experience, even when the same person consumes the same substance on different occasions. It is true that attempts have been made to delineate some patterns of effects that can be found in certain drugs. The methods through which this task has been carried out can be classified into three main approaches: structured or semistructured interviews, from which information is extracted using qualitative research methods; psychometric questionnaires, made up of a list of items that the person is asked to score according to their experience; and finally, Visual Analog Scales, or VAS. These scales are halfway between qualitative information and psychometric questionnaires and consist of a series of items such as, for example, "I liked the experience." As previously mentioned, below each one of these items there is a horizontal line of about 10 cm in length that the subject is asked to intersect at some point, making a small vertical line, depending on whether they somewhat agree (at the beginning of the horizontal line) or strongly agree (at the end of the line).

All three types of testing are generally done retrospectively. That is, in most questionnaires, participants are recruited online and asked to remember their consumption of psychedelics in general, or the last time they consumed a certain psychedelic, or another similar query, depending on each case, and answer the questionnaire based on their memory of the experience. The interviews, of course, are also carried out at some point after the consumption or consumptions. The VAS are also applied after the experience in most cases, with a few exceptions, such as the one discussed in the first chapter of this book, where study participants were asked to say a number from 1 to 100, out loud, according to the intensity of the experience they were having at that very moment.

Detailing here the entire discussion regarding the studies that have analyzed the effects of each psychedelic drug through each of these methods is entirely unrealistic. So for practical reasons, only some effects reported by psychometric questionnaires will be described, which are those that have been used systematically the most and that also allow, in many cases, a direct comparison between different studies and substances. Studies based on qualitative interviews allow us to get much closer to the subjective experience of consumers, in a more direct way and without too many intermediate analyses. They are studies that are quite easy to read, that provide verbatim fragments of transcripts of the original interviews, and that have been carried out by professionals in the social sciences, mainly experts in qualitative research. As an example, we share here an experience reported by a person who participated in a clinical trial with salvinorin-A. In this study, all the participants were asked to write up a brief report explaining their experience, although only a few isolated fragments were later published. This one in particular was previously unreleased.

From the outset, everything started very quickly. After inhalation I don't remember them reclining the bed or lowering my mask. Suddenly, after exhaling, I found myself in a space where everything was built with cubes of kaleidoscopic colors, which were rotating, moving slowly but constantly. I start to see how the walls to my right and left, with the movement of the colored cubes, are getting closer to me, and I start to worry because I feel that we have to find someone who is lost. I remember the fear of not being able to leave the room, to look for that someone. I think that during the experience I knew who it was, but at the end I couldn't remember.

I remember looking to my left and seeing Jordi and Genís [study researchers], well, guessing it was them because I also saw them in the same moving colored spheres format. Even so, I could recognize the features of their faces.

I don't remember if I talk to them, or if they say anything to me. I get the feeling that they don't pay attention to me, that they don't listen to me. But I'm not sure what to tell them either. Then, suddenly I left the scene, and I "saw" what was happening: the two researchers, me in bed . . . still seeing the colored cubes and the movement. But they were no longer approaching threateningly, they were moving and I was looking at them calmly. I was then able to relax a bit, I no longer needed to find anyone. The color visions were still there, but I no longer needed to leave, nor did I feel scared.

After a while, I started to recover bodily sensations, I noticed that I wasn't wearing the mask or the sheet over my legs, so I thought, "wow, I must have moved a lot!" and then I feel that I can't actually move yet. Already well aware of where I am, of my posture, that the experience must be ending, and I would like to move, lay on my side, but I remember being asked not to move . . . and feeling this mixture of needing to move, and not being able to do it, I feel dizzy, I have a little trouble breathing.

Jordi offers me some cool water on my face, and it makes me feel good. After a few minutes, I recovered. Oddly enough, what they tell me I have said and what they have said to me—I do not remember at all. I get the feeling that what has happened inside and what has happened outside my brain have been two completely different movies. I don't recall hearing any kind of noise or words or anything. I think the whole experience has been very visual and I kind of feel like I moved around, but I have no idea how. [Subject became very agitated as soon as the psychoactive effects appeared and intended to get up, but was calmed down and constantly reminded that she was in a study and had taken salvinorin-A. She even verbalized at some point, when she was calmer, that she understood then, that we should excuse her because she had forgotten that she had consumed a hallucinogen. However, when the effects wore off completely, she had absolutely no recollection of our conversation just a few minutes earlier.]

However, the VAS, despite being a very useful and practical tool, has not been used in such a systematic way and, furthermore, as it consists of open and flexible lists of items, different studies have selected different items, depending on the type of substance that is being studied. For example, when conducting clinical trials with salvinorin-A, it is interesting to add a VAS on "changes in dimensionality," since it seems that it tends to induce alterations in the subject's sense of dimensions. Or in the case of DMT, perhaps it is interesting to add an item about "encounters with other beings," an experience that is also common in this case. But the same items are not used in all the studies, so their comparison would not be indicated.

Data on Psychedelics' Psychoactive Effects

The most utilized questionnaires for discovering the psychoactive effects of psychedelics are: the Altered States of Consciousness or APZ (Aussergewöhnliche Psychische Zustände, according to its acronym in German) questionnaire and especially one of its later versions, the 5D-ASC (Five Dimensional-Altered States of Consciousness questionnaire); the ARCI (Addiction Research Center Inventory) questionnaire, which was specifically designed to evaluate the subjective effects and the capacity of different drugs to generate dependency; the Hallucinogen Rating Scale or HRS; and different versions of the MEQ (Mystical Experiences Questionnaire). Of all of them, only the MEQ and a later version of the APZ have reliable and robust psychometric validations. Every psychometric questionnaire must undergo various validations and complicated analyses to verify that it really measures what it is intended to measure, and that it does so in the most reliable and consistent way possible. It is a process that can take years and entails the recruitment of at least one hundred participants, in the case of questionnaires that are developed with the classical theory of tests, or more than five hundred, in the case of questionnaires developed under the item response theory, a much more complex paradigm at a mathematical level, but which is capable of designing more reliable instruments. For all these reasons, it may be understandable that many of these instruments have never been properly validated. In addition, one of the reasons why their validation has not been prioritized is because, in fact, they fulfill their function well in empirical research contexts. They are sensitive instruments, capable of discriminating between the effects of different substances (subjects administered DMT will respond differently than those administered LSD) or doses of these, showing much higher scores if the dose administered is high. What happens, however, is that, despite the fact that these questionnaires may work well from an empirical point of view, the psychopharmacology of psychedelic drugs has progressively become one of the few fields in which results are published that are apparently robust and illuminating, using questionnaires that have not been adequately validated. This, of course, is detrimental to its credibility and its reputation among experts in psychopharmacology in general, and especially among experts in psychometrics.

MEQ

The MEQ (Mystical Experiences Questionnaire) is made up of thirty items that assess the quality and intensity of mystical experiences. Some examples of items are: "experience of union with the totality," "sense of reverence," or "feelings of enjoyment," to which the person who has consumed a psychedelic substance in the past has to respond, on a scale from 0 (no, I did not experience any of this) to 5 (I lived it in an extreme way), the degree to which they feel that they experienced these sensations. The thirty items are divided into four different scales or factors: mystical, which includes unitive experiences and contact with the divine; positive mood, referring to states of ecstasy, wonder, joy, and the like; transcendence of space and time, that is, the sensation of getting out of the usual dimensions of space and time, for example, experiencing a clock minute as if it were hours or vice versa, or that physical limitations are diluted, like those that separate one's body from its environment; and finally ineffability, the inability to put words to lived experience. It would not be considered a properly mystical experience, or a complete one, if it only manifested some of these scales in an isolated way, so in order to be recognized as a truly mystical experience, it is necessary to score high on all four scales.

These four scales correspond to the usual elements of mystical experiences, which tend to be quite similar whether or not there was prior substance use. This questionnaire is focused, therefore, on the assessment of a phenomenon that can occur during the consumption of psychedelics but that is not inherent to them: the presence of mystical experiences. They tend to occur more frequently at high doses, or when the environment is also especially prone to their development (spaces with dim lighting, evocative music, natural landscapes, and the like).

The graphic representation is of great help to compare the scores obtained in this questionnaire after the consumption of different substances. This particular questionnaire has been used to study the subjective effects of psilocybin, MDMA, LSD, and 5-MeO-DMT. We can see the results in figure 34. In the case of repeated studies with the same substance, the mean obtained in each of the scales has been calculated.

It can be clearly seen that the substance that produced the highest scores on all scales was 5-MeO-DMT. In second place would be both psilocybin and LSD, with similar scores, and in last place, MDMA, which did not produce very high scores on any of the scales. This informs us of the intensity and type of effects that different substances have.

The effects of 5-MeO-DMT are characterized by abrupt onset and unusual intensity. Generally, users claim that it is more potent than DMT, producing a fairly intense experience with a strong psychological impact in the days or weeks after taking it. It is also true that it is usually consumed in ceremonial or ritual contexts, so the mystical content of the experience may just be a kind of "contamination" of the context. With LSD and psilocybin we see the presence of all four scales, although with less intensity, which is consistent with what we already know about these substances. Its effects appear much more progressively, and are also maintained for more hours, so that, in general, the experiences are less intense than in the case of 5-MeO-DMT or other psychedelics that establish psychoactive effects very abruptly, such as DMT or salvinorin-A. Finally, MDMA, as could also be deduced, does not seem to induce relevant mystical experiences. In fact, the highest score was obtained on the "positive mood" scale, probably due to the similarity between its effects and the experiences contained in the items on the scale.

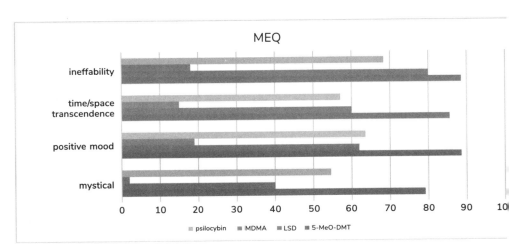

Figure 34. MEQ (Mystical Experiences Questionnaire) scores after the administration of psilocybin, MDMA, LSD, and 5-MeO-DMT in clinical trial settings. Chart prepared by the author. (See also color plate 15.)

APZ

The APZ (Altered States of Consciousness) questionnaire was specifi-cally designed to assess the type of altered state induced by different techniques, including the administration of psychedelic drugs. There are different versions available, but the most used in research is the one that contains seventy-two items and three dimensions: oceanic bound-lessness, referring to changes in the perception of time or depersonaliza-tion; dread of ego dissolution, that is, alterations in thought or control of the body associated with states of anxiety due to the loss of contact with oneself or with one's own identity; and visual restructuralization, which refers to visual distortions, synesthesia,[29] or hallucinations.

Item scoring in the APZ works in the same way as the MEQ, with the only difference being the upper limit of the scores. On the APZ, the maximum score for the oceanic boundlessness scale is 13, for the dread of ego dissolution is 22, and for the visual restructuralization scale, it is 14. This questionnaire has been used to study the effects of ayahuasca, DMT, MDE, psilocybin, and salvinorin-A.

Figure 35 shows the scores obtained using different substances. A priori, we can think that this questionnaire is less sensitive for discrim-inating between the effects of different substances, since all of them obtain quite similar scores, with the exception of psilocybin, which seems to have induced greater visual distortions and more intense oce-anic experiences in the studies. This may be due to the fact that there are few scales, and that these are also somewhat strange and not very specific. It is not very well known what constitutes an oceanic bound-lessness experience or a dread of the dissolution of the ego. If scales were used to assess more specific factors, like for visual disturbances, it would surely be possible to better discriminate between different drugs. It should be remembered that this questionnaire was designed to com-pare altered states of consciousness induced by different techniques, so it may work very well to compare states of consciousness induced with

---

29. Synesthesia is a common phenomenon in the psychedelic experience, which consists of experiencing a true crossing of sensory stimuli, so that colors can be heard or sounds can be smelled.

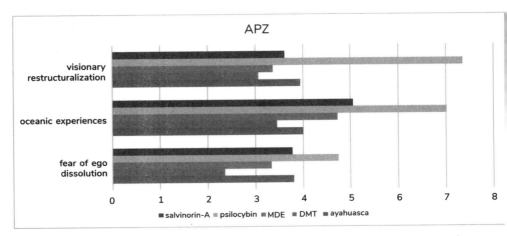

Figure 35. APZ (Altered States of Consciousness) questionnaire scores after administration of salvinorin-A, psilocybin, MDE, DMT, and ayahuasca in clinical trial settings. Chart prepared by the author. (See also color plate 16.)

the use of drugs through sensory deprivation and with the use of the shamanic drum. But perhaps it does not work as well to compare the state of consciousness induced by different psychedelics.

HRS

The HRS (Hallucinogen Rating Scale) questionnaire was developed by Dr. Rick Strassman, one of the pioneers of psychedelic drug research, especially in the "psychedelic renaissance" that has occurred since the 1990s. It consists of seventy-one items grouped into six scales or factors that can be altered after the consumption of psychedelic drugs: somesthesia, which includes somatic or physical effects; affective, referring to emotional or affective responses; perception, which measures visual, auditory, gustatory, or olfactory alterations; cognition, which includes modifications in the process or contents of thought; volition, which describes the subject's ability to voluntarily interact with himself or with the environment; and lastly, intensity, which, as the name suggests, reflects the overall intensity of the experience.

The scores work in the same way as in previous cases, and this is perhaps one of the best examples of an instrument that works well empirically but whose theoretical structure has not been confirmed by the few psychometric analyses carried out to date, so that improved versions have been proposed. However, to date, the original questionnaire is still used, although there is less and less research that includes it, precisely because of its poor psychometric properties.

The HRS has been used in studies where ayahuasca, DMT, ketamine, salvinorin-A, MDMA, and psilocybin have been administered. Figure 36 shows the different patterns of effects obtained. At first glance, MDMA and psilocybin are the substances that got the highest scores on various scales. However, this does not necessarily reflect the reality of the effects that these substances tend to produce. Other variables can influence the results, and consideration of these other variables is essential in the psychopharmacology of psychedelics. As has often been pointed out in this book, we are constantly talking about complex phenomena, and the evaluation of the psychoactive effects of different substances does not escape this rule.

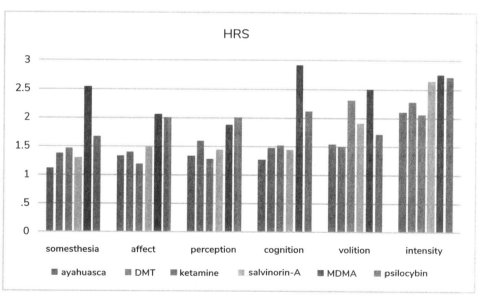

Figure 36. HRS (Hallucinogen Rating Scale) questionnaire scores after administration of ayahuasca, DMT, ketamine, salvinorin-A, MDMA, and psilocybin in clinical trial settings. Chart prepared by the author. (See also color plate 17.)

In this case, for example, not all studies used the same doses, and even using the same doses, the methods of administration were not equally effective. This is the case for salvinorin-A, for example. The data from some studies in which the method of administration was completely ineffective were not reflected, of course, but even so, among the studies that did manage to administer the substance quite well, there were also notable differences in subjective experience. It seems that the place where salvinorin-A was administered most effectively was at the Hospital de la Santa Creu i Sant Pau, in Barcelona, where the subjects were previously trained to perform an uninterrupted aspiration of thirty seconds or more, during which the researchers caused the vaporization of crystallized salvinorin-A.

The previous experience of the subjects or their own physical or psychological characteristics also have a great influence. In the case of MDMA, for example, the only study in which the HRS was conducted was in a clinical trial of women suffering treatment-resistant PTSD and without prior experience with MDMA, so the experience must have been very intense for them compared to people with previous experience, as in fact happens in a large part of the clinical trials with psychedelics, as mentioned above. In fact, high scores on the volition scale indicate a disruption in the ability to interact with the environment, something that is characteristically seen in high doses of salvinorin-A, after which the subjects not only cannot answer questions asked by the researchers, but they don't even remember what happened in those few minutes, so they can move, scream, and kick, and then remember nothing at all. This situation is unlikely to occur after administering MDMA, although, as we see in figure 36, MDMA has a higher score than salvinorin-A.

5D-ASC

As we have commented in the first paragraphs of this section, the 5D-ASC (Five Dimensional-Altered States of Consciousness) questionnaire is a later version of the APZ, so it contains some of its scales (oceanic boundlessness, visual restructuralization, and dread

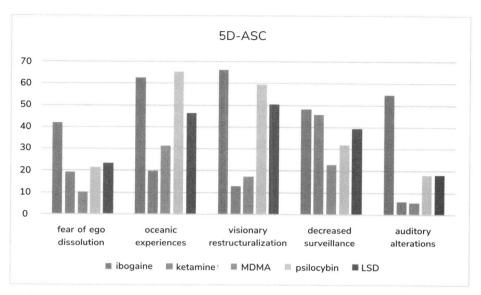

Figure 37. The 5D-ASC (Five Dimensional-Altered States of Consciousness) questionnaire scores after administration of ibogaine, ketamine, MDMA, psilocybin, and LSD in clinical trial settings. Chart prepared by the author. (See also color plate 18.)

of ego dissolution), in addition to two others: reduction of vigilance (referring to clouding of consciousness or numbness) and auditory alterations.

The questionnaire contains ninety-four items and has been widely used to study the effects of LSD, psilocybin, MDMA, ibogaine, and ketamine. It is perhaps the most widely used questionnaire today and the one that seems to be gaining even more importance due to the psychometric analyses to which it has been subjected. Figure 37 shows a comparison between the effects recorded after administering different psychedelic drugs. Ibogaine shows high scores on all scales, while ketamine and MDMA show rather low scores. Psilocybin, however, shows high scores especially on the "ocean boundlessness" and "visual restructuralization" scales. These data may suggest that this questionnaire, despite the fact that it has been widely used in ketamine research, may be especially indicated when classic psychedelics are used.

Tolerance

We cannot speak of psychoactive effects without speaking, at least briefly, about the phenomenon of tolerance. Tolerance is defined as desensitization to the effects of a drug or substance, that is, the drug loses its effect, and it is necessary to increase the dose to achieve the same effects. This becomes very evident in the case of the psychoactive effects of psychedelic drugs. After the administration of a single dose, there is a marked tolerance that causes the effects of that same dose to be significantly attenuated if it is consumed again over the following days.

The mechanism underlying this desensitization is the physiological response of the 5-HT2A receptor to its potent activation by most psychedelics. This strong stimulation causes a process called "downregulation" of this receptor. This means that the number of 5-HT2A receptors is reduced, so that if the body is subjected to a new dose before this downregulation disappears, the effect it produces will be much less, since far fewer receptors will be available to "collect" the substance's molecules. It is generally assumed that between three and seven days after the use of a psychedelic drug, the density of 5-HT2A receptors returns to 50 percent of what it was before use, a density that is already functional for sensing most of the effects, although it is advisable to wait about two more weeks so that the density of receptors is the same as before the first consumption.

It should be noted that tolerance does not only occur when some drugs are used repeatedly, such as taking LSD on Monday and using it again on Wednesday. It also occurs between psychedelics of different classes, for example between simple tryptamines and phenethylamines. Using the same example, if you take LSD on Monday and mescaline on Wednesday, the mescaline will have far less effect. The same would happen with psilocybin or any psychedelic whose main mechanism of action is the activation of the 5-HT2A receptor. When tolerance between different drugs occurs, we speak of cross-tolerance.

Both tolerance and cross-tolerance are thought to play a certain protective role against the eventual development of addictive behaviors.

While it is true that psychedelic-inducing experiences are not usually habit forming and these are not deliberately sought, experiencing them often and the speed at which tolerance is reached by these substances also prevents the abuse of psychedelics. This is mainly because, if compulsive consumption were to occur, they would immediately cease to have an effect, and there would be no physiological or psychological response that could act as a reinforcer.

Interestingly, although it has always been thought that DMT does not produce tolerance, this statement needs some nuancing. A recent study found acute tolerance effects in continuous intravenous infusions of DMT, so that the effects appear to remain stable between thirty and ninety minutes after administration, regardless of variations caused in systemic circulation.[30] Previous studies did not report tolerance effects after different intermittent administrations of intravenous DMT, so perhaps the absence of tolerance can be observed after administrations separated in time, but not in a context of continuous administration. Salvinorin-A, as already mentioned, seems to not produce tolerance, although it is rare for users of salvinorin-A to want to repeat the experience, especially when high doses are used.

REFERENCES FOR FURTHER STUDY

Aday JS, Davis AK, Mitzkovitz CM, Bloesch EK, Davoli CC. 2021. Predicting reactions to psychedelic drugs: a systematic review of states and traits related to acute drug effects. ACS Pharmacology & Translational Science 4(2):424–435.

Bouso JC, Pedrero-Pérez EJ, Gandy S, Alcázar-Córcoles MÁ. 2016. Measuring the subjective: revisiting the psychometric properties of three rating scales that assess the acute effects of hallucinogens. Human Psychopharmacology 31(5):356–372.

Breeksema JJ, Kuin BW, Kamphuis J, van den Brink W, Vermetten E, Schoevers RA. 2022. Adverse events in clinical treatments with serotonergic

---

30. Vogt SB, Ley L, Erne L, et al. 2023. Acute effects of intravenous DMT in a randomized placebo-controlled study in healthy participants. Translational Psychiatry 13(172).

psychedelics and MDMA: a mixed-methods systematic review. Journal of Psychopharmacology 36(10):1100–1117.

Brunton LL, editor. 2018. Goodman & Gilman's: the pharmacological basis of therapeutics. 13th ed. New York (NY): McGraw-Hill Education.

Calvey T, Howells FM. 2018. An introduction to psychedelic neuroscience. Progress in Brain Research 242:1–23.

Casarotto PC, Girych M, Fred SM, Kovaleva V, Moliner R, Enkavi G, Biojone C, Cannarozzo C, Sahu MP, Kaurinkoski K, et al. 2021. Antidepressant drugs act by directly binding to TRKB neurotrophin receptors. Cell 184(5):1299–1313.

Dos Santos RG, Bouso JC, Alcázar-Córcoles MÁ, Hallak J. 2018. Efficacy, tolerability, and safety of serotonergic psychedelics for the management of mood, anxiety, and substance-use disorders: a systematic review of systematic reviews. Expert Review of Clinical Pharmacology 11(9):889–902.

Elsey JWB. 2017. Psychedelic drug use in healthy individuals: a review of benefits, costs, and implications for drug policy. Drug Science, Policy and Law, doi.org/10.1177/2050324517723232.

Flanagan TW, Nichols CD. 2018. Psychedelics as anti-inflammatory agents. International Review of Psychiatry 30(4):363–375.

Halberstadt AL. 2015. Recent advances in the neuropsychopharmacology of serotonergic hallucinogens. Behavioral Brain Research 277:99–120.

Hartogsohn I. 2018. The meaning-enhancing properties of psychedelics and their mediator role in psychedelic therapy, spirituality, and creativity. Frontiers in Neuroscience 12:129.

Kozlowska U, Nichols C, Wiatr K, Figiel M. 2022. From psychiatry to neurology: psychedelics as prospective therapeutics for neurodegenerative disorders. Journal of Neurochemistry 162(1):89–108.

Leonard JB, Anderson B, Klein-Schwartz W. 2018. Does getting high hurt?: characterization of cases of LSD and psilocybin-containing mushroom exposures to national poison centers between 2000 and 2016. Journal of Psychopharmacology 32(12):1286–1294.

Liechti ME, Holze F. 2022. Dosing psychedelics and MDMA. Current Topics in Behavioral Neurosciences 56:3–21.

Moliner R, Girych M, Brunello CA, et al. 2023. Psychedelics promote plasticity by directly binding to BDNF receptor TrkB. Nature Neuroscience 26(6):1032–1041.

Nielson EM, Guss J. 2018. The influence of therapists' first-hand experience with psychedelics on psychedelic-assisted psychotherapy research and therapist training. Journal of Psychedelic Studies 2(2):64–73.

Olson DE. 2018. Psychoplastogens: a promising class of plasticity-promoting neurotherapeutics. Journal of Experimental Neuroscience 12:1179069518800508.

Riba J, Valle M, Urbano G, Yritia M, Morte A, Barbanoj MJ. 2003. Human pharmacology of ayahuasca: subjective and cardiovascular effects, monoamine metabolite excretion, and pharmacokinetics. The Journal of Pharmacology and Experimental Therapeutics 306(1):73–83.

Riba J, McIlhenny EH, Bouso JC, Barker SA. 2015. Metabolism and urinary disposition of N,N- dimethyltryptamine after oral and smoked administration: a comparative study. Drug Testing and Analysis 7(5):401–406.

Shafiee A, Arabzadeh Bahri R, Rafiei MA, et al. 2024. The effect of psychedelics on the level of brain-derived neurotrophic factor: a systematic review and meta-analysis. Journal of Psychopharmacology.

Singh JA. 2021. Epidemiology of hospitalizations with hallucinogen use disorder: a 17-year US national study. Journal of Addictive Diseases 39(4):545–549.

Vollenweider FX, Smallridge JW. 2022. Classic psychedelic drugs: update on biological mechanisms. Pharmacopsychiatry 55(3):121–138.

Zamberlan F, Sanz C, Martínez Vivot R, Pallavicini C, Erowid F, Erowid E, Tagliazucchi E. 2018. The varieties of the psychedelic experience: a preliminary study of the association between the reported subjective effects and the binding affinity profiles of substituted phenethylamines and tryptamines. Frontiers in Integrative Neuroscience 12:54.

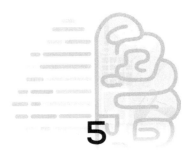

5

Harm Reduction in Your Use of Psychedelic Drugs

Disease research has advanced so much that it is increasingly difficult to find someone who is completely healthy.

ALDOUS HUXLEY

From the pharmacological point of view, there are some aspects that can help reduce the risk of developing adverse reactions associated with the use of psychedelics. Most of these strategies have been implemented, in one way or another, in clinical trials or experimental research, but they can also be used in the event that an adult decides to consume a substance. We must reiterate, at this point, that this book is not intended to promote the consumption of legal or illegal substances and, in fact, we do not recommend that anyone approach these drugs unless it is in a clinical space and accompanied by health professionals, be it medicine or psychology. It should also be noted that, although we can describe how these substances affect some receptors or the functioning of some systems, we still do not know much about how they work, especially with regard to consciousness, information processing, or the content and dynamics of thought, so the wisest thing would be to refrain from experiences with still unknown effects. If someone still decides to consume, at least reduce the possible risks as much as possible in the following ways.

Take Care of Yourself

In clinical trials and in many other contexts, somewhat more implicitly, this point is insisted upon. Subjects are asked to get eight hours of sleep, to avoid arriving stressed or running, to take their time, to try to refrain from drinking alcohol in the previous days, and to have a light breakfast. All these tips can be summed up in the advice: "take care of yourself."

When you want to use psychedelics, you want your body to be in perfect condition, so you can enjoy the experience with less chance of ending up exhausted or disoriented. This includes not consuming when you have a cold, the flu, a COVID-19 variant, or if you haven't slept for a day or two. These experiences can be especially strenuous for both the brain and the body in general, so it is best to plan carefully and find a space and time when you feel well and can spend the necessary time to experiment safely.

Check What You Bought

In Spain and other countries there are organizations such as Spain's Energy Control[1] or DanceSafe[2] that analyze a wide range of substances free of charge, or at a low price, to check their purity or the presence of possible adulterants. It is a basic risk reduction strategy that is becoming more and more widespread in different countries and contexts. To act in an informed way, consumers must first be informed. Unfortunately, there are still many countries where there is no way (or at least no easy or affordable way) to do this, so perhaps this is not a recommendation applicable to all readers of this book. However, those who have the possibility should always analyze the substances they are going to consume.

In the case of psilocybin mushrooms, for example, there is not much risk, because there are few possibilities of adulteration, but as far as LSD or other substances are concerned, it is common for them to be adulterated or even replaced by completely different substances. This is the case

1. A nonprofit organization focused on harm reduction and drug education. Founded in the 1990s, it aims to provide accurate information, support, and advice to drug users to promote safer use and minimize the risks associated with drug consumption.
2. DanceSafe is a nonprofit organization that promotes health and safety within the electronic music and dance community.

with DOC or AL-LAD, which are often sold as LSD, for example, and can be much more toxic and carry more risks. MDMA or ketamine, depending on the format, can also be easily doctored. Even when there are no illicit intentions there can be confusion, so, for one reason or another, it is always advisable to analyze a sample of what you want to consume.

Don't Get Creative with Routes of Administration

If something works, why change it? It is one of the basic lessons that can be learned from evolutionary biology and one of the tips that we have to highlight here. From MDMA by the anus to LSD cartons in the eyes, there's a whole motley collection of bizarre and potentially dangerous routes of administration that were either all the rage at one point or are still practiced in some consumer circles.

Few, if any, of these alternative routes make sense from a pharmacological point of view. The body has been used, for millions of years, to ingest many types of exogenous matter, be it an apple or a mushroom, orally. It is the safest way to do it. The substance will begin to be absorbed through the saliva and then in the gastrointestinal tract, reaching the liver and kidneys and following its normal course. Other routes of administration are often justified on the grounds that there are mucous membranes on the eyelid, rectum, or vagina that rapidly absorb the substance in question. And it is true, the substance is going to be absorbed by those places, but this will only complicate the whole process. We have a beautiful and

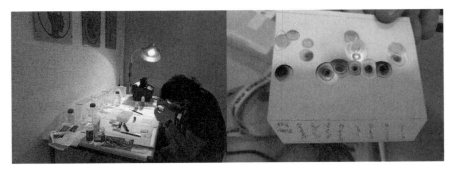

Figure 38. Analysis of substances in ISOLAb, founded by the Associació Reus Som Útils (ARSU), one of the pioneering organizations in the field of risk and harm reduction. Images courtesy of Antoniu Llort.

extensive mucosa in the mouth; we do not need to explore other avenues. Sublingual absorption is fast and effective, at least equal to, if not more absorbent than, other mucous membranes.

It's okay to want to cross borders and explore unknown territories, but in some things it's better to settle for traditional wisdom. If a substance has always been consumed in a certain way, follow suit.

Keep Hydrated

Hydration is essential, but don't overdo it either. Remember the case of MDMA, described above. Nevertheless, it is always a good idea to maintain good hydration. Particularly with LSD, due to its long-lasting effects, but also with other psychedelics, hunger is usually reduced. While you are under the influence of a psychedelic, and perhaps for a while longer, eating is something you will not even consider, except perhaps for some sweets or fruits, whose taste you might enjoy even more.

Precisely because we are immersed in a trip where any stimulus is worthy of excessive attention, we can go hours without eating or drinking and we won't even realize it. That is why, sometimes, headaches or other symptoms may appear, but not as a direct consequence of consumption, but rather due to dehydration or lack of electrolytes.[3] In these cases, it is recommended to leave several glasses of water in safe places, that cannot fall or be tripped over, but that are "close at hand," so that they are easy to access. As long as we maintain hydration, the body will suffer less from any demanding situation to which we subject it.

Don't Mix

It is always a good idea to consume psychedelics without mixing them with other substances. This is recommended not only because their effects will be experienced in a "cleaner" way, allowing you to become

---

3. Electrolytes, such as sodium and potassium, are necessary for adequate cell operation and communication. When sodium levels are low, for example, you can enter a state of hyponatremia, mentioned in a previous chapter regarding the risks of MDMA.

familiar with the particular effects, but also to avoid the potential consequences of dangerous interactions.

The main risk of interaction between psychedelic drugs and other substances or drugs is related to the inhibition or induction of their metabolism through liver enzymes that we have seen in previous chapters. In this sense, it is important to know the enzymes (CYPs) that metabolize the substance that we are taking and those that metabolize other substances or medications with which we want to mix it, understanding that, if these are the same, it is a bad idea to mix. This could lead to intoxication or to experiencing the psychoactive effects of psychedelics for a longer period of time. For example, beta-carbolines in ayahuasca are processed by CYP2D6. If the person who wants to consume ayahuasca is taking paroxetine or fluoxetine, two widely used antidepressants that are powerful inhibitors of the CYP2D6 enzyme, they could suffer from intoxication by beta-carbolines, with symptoms like dizziness, vomiting (more than usual), ataxia, and other muscular symptoms, as well as alterations in blood pressure.

Another risk that is often mentioned in the consumption of psychedelics is what is known as "serotonergic syndrome," when these substances are mixed with antidepressants or other drugs that increase serotonin levels, such as the pain medication tramadol. Abnormally high levels of serotonin cause symptoms that may start out mildly, as occurs in the case of taking SSRI-type antidepressants, which produce symptoms such as nausea, diarrhea, or insomnia (while not combined with other substances), or more severely in cases, above all, in which a combination of medications or substances causes symptoms such as muscle stiffness, delirium, and very extreme variations in blood pressure, possibly even leading to coma or death.

Some cases of fatalities have been reported, especially with the use of MDMA and 5-MeO-DMT when these have been combined with drugs or other substances that also increase serotonin levels. Other cases of fatalities associated with the use of ayahuasca or other substances could also be attributed to this syndrome, although a clear direct relationship has not been demonstrated in all cases. One of the fundamental problems that limit prevention and possible intervention in cases of serotonergic syndrome is that some of its symptoms are, in fact, common effects reported by users, such as symptoms of delirium, tremors, and dysregulation of body temperature. Therefore, it is not always possible to act in time, even when there are people in charge of supervising or caring for consumers.

However, it is not enough to have this information about liver enzymes or to avoid the combination of substances that increase serotonin levels. These are just some of the more common interactions, but there are many other mechanisms by which dangerous interactions can occur. Therefore, from the outset, the best strategy is not to mix anything. If you are taking medications for some important indications that do not allow a safe interruption of the medication, it is recommended to check possible interactions with your family doctor, trusted pharmacist, or through some services that have been recently implemented, given the need for this type of advice.

Be Patient

Especially when taking MDMA, but generally when taking any psychedelic, it is important to wait a reasonable time before taking another dose. Most psychedelics are taken orally, so their effects can take a long time to manifest. In addition, the first effects are subtle, so it may be difficult to recognize them until they are especially noticeable. A good way to check if you are already under the effects of a psychedelic drug is to observe physical manifestations. Take a pen or any other object and see if you tremble when you hold it (if there is a slight tremor, it means that the substance is already acting) or observe your pupils and see if they are larger than normal (mydriasis).

In any case, possible additional doses should be reserved for at least two to two and a half hours after consumption. And if you have been able to analyze the substance and know perfectly well the dose you have taken, you might wait to experience some more, or settle for a calm and peaceful experience, so that you can increase the dose a bit more another day until you achieve the desired effects. There is no hurry.

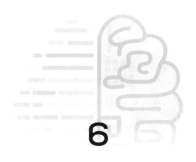

6

A Look into the Future
Promises and Challenges

Truth is not what is demonstrable, but what is inescapable.
ANTOINE DE SAINT-EXUPÉRY

I have never liked predictions or forecasts, precisely because they almost never come true. They also tend to inform more about the person who states them than about the reality they are supposedly talking about. The objective of this last section is not to predict or imagine a near future that no one knows will come true, but I would like to discuss some aspects of the current research with psychedelic drugs that *are already happening*, and that will surely have implications into the future. This perspective is a personal one. Others would surely highlight different aspects, so the following paragraphs should not be taken as concerns generally present in the field of psychedelic research, a field that, like most others, is broad, diverse, and heterogeneous enough for divergent opinions and points of view.

MARKETING OF PSYCHEDELIC THERAPIES

At the time of this writing (early 2022), both psilocybin and MDMA are in phase III clinical trials; that is, the last of the phases prior to commercialization. It is therefore very likely that during 2024 or at some point in 2025, psychotherapies assisted with these drugs will already have been approved by the Food and Drug Administration (FDA) or the European Medicines Agency (EMA) (regulatory agencies of the United States and Europe, respectively, in charge of authorizing the marketing of new drugs).

The availability of these treatments will have to be accompanied by adequate contexts for their psychotherapeutic development. It is likely that as soon as this authorization is obtained there will be a significant proliferation of centers where this will be carried out. It is still unlikely that public health systems will be able to assume the practice of these psychotherapies as something habitual, since these require two therapists and therapeutic support before and after each session, as well as, of course, much more frequent visits to the psychologist. In Spain, for example, visits to a psychologist through the public health system are usually limited to one hour a month (if you're lucky). The kind of preparation and therapeutic alliance that psychedelic-assisted psychotherapy requires simply cannot be generated in the relationship that is established with a therapist whom one visits once a month. This makes us think that, at least for several years, these treatments will be limited to private clinics. In a private clinic you will surely be able to find the space and time necessary to carry out the treatment safely, although of course this will also lead to unaffordable costs for the vast majority of patients.

According to a report from the United States Census Bureau,[1] 11.5 percent of the North American population is living at the poverty line. What is more remarkable is that the population with fewer economic resources is at special risk of developing mental disorders such as depression or anxiety.[2] Therefore, with the restriction of psychedelic-assisted psychotherapies to private clinics, an important sector of the population

---

1. United States Census Bureau. 2023. Poverty in the United States: 2022. Retrieved from U.S. Census Bureau website.
2. Ridley MW, Rao G, Schilbach F, Patel VH. 2020. Poverty, depression, and anxiety: causal evidence and mechanisms. Working Paper Series No. 27157. Cambridge (MA): National Bureau of Economic Research.

that could benefit from these treatments, but unfortunately will not be able to afford them, will be abandoned. This clashes directly with the supposed feelings of uniqueness, empathy, and compassion that the psychedelic experience itself tends to evoke, which is likely to place therapists and patients in an admittedly complicated and paradoxical position. Patient groups and some institutions will surely have to fight to enforce their rights (remember that the right to health is one of the fundamental rights of human beings) and perhaps mechanisms will be found that can guarantee that at least a percentage of treatments in these clinics will be intended for people with an unfavorable economic or social situation.

Another aspect for which we must be prepared is the possibility that these treatments may be applied in other conditions for which they were not initially approved. This happens with many medications and is often referred to as "off-label" prescription. When regulatory agencies authorize the marketing of a drug, they also do so for a specific condition or illness. In other words, a drug is not approved "in general," but rather for a specific purpose. However, once drugs are approved, they can be prescribed for other diseases besides the original one, as long as there is sufficient theoretical or clinical information to justify such a prescription. It is a somewhat risky move, because if serious adverse reactions occur when the drug is prescribed for the medical condition for which it was approved, the responsibility falls on the regulatory agency or the pharmaceutical company, depending on the case. However, the responsibility for adverse reactions occurring in "off-label" prescriptions is assumed by the prescribing physician. Even so, this type of prescription is quite common in clinical practice, so we can expect that psychotherapies assisted with MDMA or psilocybin will end up being applied, in the near future, to a wide range of physical and mental illnesses, potentially offering interesting data and clues for very promising future uses currently unidentified.

THE ROLE OF TRADITIONAL KNOWLEDGE

A story that has been repeated ad nauseum in science is that of the appropriation of plants and traditional remedies by academics from all kinds of disciplines, from botany to pharmacology. Generally, the story consists of white men visiting "Third World" countries (the Global South, or whatever name you want to give to countries with high poverty rates), who discover that the local populations use some particular plant or product for the alleviation of a specific symptom or disease. White men take samples of this product, analyze it in their laboratories, isolate some of its active ingredients, patent them, market them, and make millions in annual profits, while completely forgetting about the people who surely provided them altruistically with all the information that they possessed on the product (accumulated and perfected over generations). It is also common that the indications for which these drugs, discovered thanks to traditional knowledge, are prescribed are also widely present among the local population from which the plant or product in question was originally extracted. So, paradoxically, people will continue to die or suffer in these places because they do not have access to the medicine that was discovered thanks to them.

Recent events in research with psychedelics seem to indicate that history is repeating itself. This is because no reciprocity mechanism has yet been implemented to compensate and thank the original peoples for the discoveries that they themselves contributed to, such as the use of psilocybin mushrooms, ayahuasca, and ibogaine. Moreover, there are truly regrettable stories, such as the terrible events related to María Sabina, the medicine woman of the Mazatec people thanks to whom Albert Hofmann was finally able to identify and isolate psilocybin, or the scarcity of plants for the preparation of ayahuasca that already has begun in some Amazonian regions.

It seems that the marketing of these substances for therapeutic use will be carried out by private for-profit companies, so it is unlikely that part of the profits will be donated to local communities in countries such as Mexico, Peru, Brazil, and Gabon. However, we face not only an ethical problem but also a scientific and epistemological one. As has already been stated in this book, the use of natural products can be more beneficial compared to the use of their active ingredients. This is what is proposed from polypharmacology, the last of the paradigms that emerged in pharmacology and that is revolutionizing the foundations of the discipline. In the case of psychedelics, as we have mentioned before, this translates into the possibility that the use of psilocybin mushrooms is safer and more effective than the use of its isolated active ingredients, the same occurring in the case of ayahuasca and other products. However, the use of these natural products instead of their active ingredients could not be patented in any way, and nobody would benefit. So the marketing of active ingredients by pharmaceutical companies would not only be threatening the value of traditional knowledge, which would not be rewarded at any time, but would also be acting against the same scientific principles that state that it would be much more advantageous to work with completely natural products. Fortunately, there are already some initiatives in Mexico and Israel that are betting on research with standardized extracts of *Psilocybe* mushrooms. In particular, a study recently published found that the *Psilocybe* extract had a more potent and prolonged effect on synaptic plasticity than psilocybin.[3]

Given this scenario, it is likely that in the not-so-distant future many people will seek these treatments in more informal contexts. In fact, although these substances are not yet approved for clinical use, there has been a fairly extensive network of therapists for many years, both in the United States and Europe, as well as in other regions, who apply the psychedelic-assisted psychotherapy model in a clandestine and discreet way. These treatments may not only be more affordable but may even work better, precisely because they make use of whole natural products. Again, we are obtaining preliminary evidence that suggests such products may have an advantageous profile compared to isolated molecules. This could be a much more community-based model that coexists with the private clinic model, although some type of self-regulation process must also be carried out to guarantee minimum security criteria, good

---

3. Shahar O, Botvinnik A, Shwartz A, et al. 2024. Effect of chemically synthesized psilocybin and psychedelic mushroom extract on molecular and metabolic profiles in mouse brain. Molecular Psychiatry.

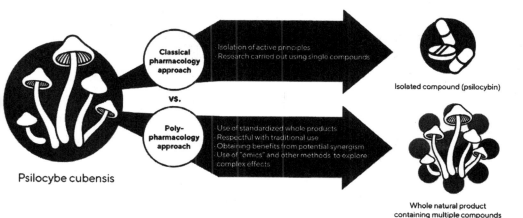

Figure 39. Example of the application of the classical pharmacology paradigm (*upper* arrow) or the polypharmacology paradigm (*lower* arrow) in the clinical development of psilocybin mushrooms. In the classical paradigm, the active ingredients, in this case psilocybin, are isolated and purified, and all the studies are carried out with this compound. In the case of polypharmacology, standardized extracts of the product are made, that is, products that contain psilocybin but also all the other components of the mushrooms, ensuring that their proportion is always the same. This approach is respectful and aligned with traditional knowledge, as it follows its guidelines more faithfully; certain benefits are obtained at the level of pharmacology, such as the display of synergy between the compounds of the mushrooms, which can end up producing much more powerful effects; and it allows the use of techniques developed in recent years to analyze and identify complex effects of natural products. Original image appeared in the article: Ona G, Dos Santos RG, Hallak JEC, Bouso JC. 2020. Polypharmacology or "pharmacological promiscuity" in psychedelic research: what are we missing? ACS Chemical Neuroscience 11(20):3191–3193. Reproduced with the authors' permission.

practices, prevention of intrusion, respect, and possible compensation mechanisms and protection of these practices in traditional contexts.

TO TRIP OR NOT TO TRIP

As psychedelic research moves forward, it is likely that new indications and uses for different psychedelic drugs will be approved. This broad spectrum of possibilities increasingly limits the induction of powerful hallucinogenic effects. Despite seeming like an attractive experience to some people, we must not forget, as it has already been mentioned in this book, that only 1 to 2 percent of the population have had experiences with psychedelic drugs. These drugs do not attract a large number of users, as the drugs tend to be associated with madness, loss of control, hallucinations, or with people who have been left "unhinged." Therefore, it is to be expected that the number of patients willing to enter a psychedelic trip to solve their problems are rather few.

In this sense, work is already being done with analogs of DMT, salvinorin-A, psilocybin, and other compounds that are not psychoactive but that can induce, it seems, the same benefits. In fact, some animal studies have already shown antidepressant effects of psilocybin and LSD independently from their 5-HT2A receptor agonists.[4] Therefore, a scenario in which nonpsychoactive compounds can be synthesized that could still be more effective than current psychiatric drugs is beginning to be plausible. Other applications for which some psychedelics are being investigated are rehabilitation after strokes and the prevention of the development of neurodegenerative diseases. In these cases, the induction of hallucinogenic effects would not be desirable either.

This raises the question of the extent to which subjective experience is necessary for psychedelics to have therapeutic effects. Perhaps they could be turned into pills that are taken every six to eight hours, like aspirin or paracetamol, which, from a somewhat more romantic perspective, would imply that a certain "magic" would be lost, together with certain learning and special experiences that usually accompany any therapeutic changes made with psychedelic drugs. Perhaps many patients are not interested in accessing transpersonal realities, or having metaphysical or spiritual experiences, or even coming into direct contact with their biographical or family past. Perhaps they simply want to stop suffering, lead a normal life, be able to go to work, and so forth. For

---

4. You can consult the following article to delve deeper into this issue: Service RF. 2022. Psychedelics without hallucinations? Science (New York, NY) 375(6579):370.

them, perhaps, a nonpsychoactive derivative of psilocybin or any other psychedelic would be more appropriate. Some of the benefits may be lost, of course, but it is better to lose these than the patients themselves.

What is clear, and what we can take away from this, is that we should not be closed off to future options for ideological, political, or moral reasons, which are already involved in scientific research, since many groups have clearly and resoundingly positioned themselves in the defense (or not) of the subjective effects of psychedelics. We think that this attitude is in fact unscientific and more so when considering patients suffering from mental disorders who already have enough with their condition to have to face dogmatic and incomprehensible positions. They should be able to choose what is most appropriate for them. Science, for its part, should limit itself to doing the same to ensure that these different possibilities can be offered.

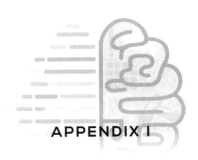

The Legal Status of Psychedelic Drugs around the World

Francisco Azorín Ortega is a lawyer specializing in legislation and jurisprudence on drugs. The information in this appendix is as up-to-date as possible as of this writing. This information is subject to change.

I. INTRODUCTION

In order to talk about legislation and jurisprudence on psychedelic drugs, the first thing we have to do is define the latter concept. Although depending on how broadly the term is interpreted it may have different meanings, on this occasion we will use a fairly broad definition of the term. Such definition will include all those substances such as LSD, DMT, psilocybin, mescaline, and 2C-B that have perceptible effects on consciousness through, noticeably, acting on the serotonin 2A neuroreceptors, as well as other substances with more dissociative psychedelic effects, such as ketamine, which acts mainly on NMDA glutamate neuroreceptors. There are also other substances classified as empathogenic-entactogenic, such as MDMA ("ecstasy"), with indirect interaction on serotonin 2A neuroreceptors, which many consider to be only semipsychedelic, but which in high doses can cause considerable psychedelic effects, like those caused by its sister substance, MDA[1], or 2C-B.

It should also be noted that these psychedelic drugs can occur as isolated molecules (either extracted or synthesized), or as part of a plant or fungus (ayahuasca, psilocybe mushrooms, cacti, and the like), or even in some animals, such as the toad *Bufo alvarius* from the Sonoran Desert (Mexico), whose glands contain the most potent of the known psychedelics, 5-MeO-DMT. Although these toads were only recently discovered to contain this molecule, 5-MeO-DMT had already been synthesized in 1936 and isolated in 1959 from the seeds of the South American tree *Anadenanthera colubrina*. Another drug that is also found in animals is DMT. On top of being present in many plants, this molecule is also found in small amounts in humans and other mammals. It, therefore, seems that these compounds may be far more important to the workings of nature than we could ever have imagined.

Today, the Western world has far more psychedelics at its disposal than could have been available in the psychedelic boom era of the 1960s and 1970s, as well as in the "Second Summer of Love," which took place in Ibiza in 1987 and was exported to the United Kingdom between 1988 and 1989 with the emergence of the semipsychedelic MDMA and "rave culture."

The explosion of the phenomenon of new designer drugs, new psychoactive substances (NPS), and their sale on the internet, as well as the growing interest in shamanic cultures and their practice in Western territories, make it necessary to review and clarify the legislation and jurisprudence that tries to deal with this social reality. The presence of a certain sector of the population that uses these substances on an occasional or recurrent basis to navigate their consciousness, reconcile and accept their traumas, free themselves from their blockages, relieve their stress or depression, and, in short, try to live in this increasingly confrontational society more consciously and peacefully is becoming increasingly evident in our current culture.

---

1. It was known in the popular slang of Spain in the 1980s and 1990s as "mescalinas" or "meskas" because of the similarity between its structure and some of its effects to those of mescaline, found in the San Pedro cactus and Mexican peyote.

The legal regime for psychedelic drugs around the world is a complex subject that has always been given to controversy and disparate interpretations, as well as constant legislative changes. In this appendix, I will attempt to provide as comprehensive and up-to-date a review as possible.

1.1 Why Were Certain Psychoactive Substances Banned?

The idea of banning all "recreational" use of certain psychoactive substances was driven by the growing influence of Anglo-American Christian Puritanism and the temperance movement against alcohol in the late 19th and early 20th centuries, which in the United States also led to the prohibition of alcohol between 1920 and 1933. The campaign for prohibition was also fuelled by racist sentiments towards immigrants from China and Mexico, who used opium and cannabis.[2]

In the 1960s, specifically in 1961, most countries in the world signed the Single Convention on Narcotic Drugs in New York, which banned opium, cannabis, and coca leaf, as well as their active ingredients and some derivatives (cocaine, morphine, and heroin). Later, new trends in the use of psychoactive drugs would emerge, such as the popularization of psychedelic substances, given that, in parallel to the promising clinical research with substances like LSD, psilocybin, and mescaline, some university professors such as Timothy Leary, writers such as Ken Kesey, and actors such as Cary Grant made their use fashionable in North America. This meant that the use of this category of substances quickly spread to the rest of the Western world, also playing an important role in the development of modern neuroscience.

With the upsurge of the nonclinical use of LSD, DMT, and psilocybin in the 1960s, associated with the hippie movement, the counterculture, and opposition to the Vietnam War, as well as their use in relation to some events reported in a very sensationalist way by the

---

2. Arbour, et al. 2019. Classification of psychoactive substances. Geneva (Switzerland): Global Commission on Drug Policy. Report 2019. Retrieved from the Global Commission on Drug Policy website.

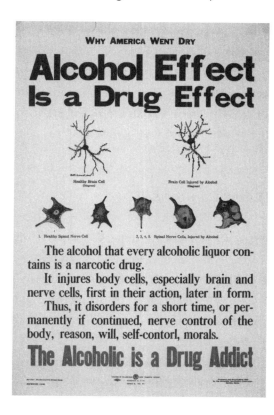

Figure 40. The scientific temperance movement against alcohol, which had a strong Puritan influence, enacted alcohol prohibition in the United States. Image by The Scientific Temperance Foundation.

press, at the end of the decade, the United States decided to ban these substances. The first to do so was the state of California in 1966 when Ronald Reagan was governor, and they were later controlled at the federal level in 1969. Subsequently, in 1971, they were included in Schedule I of the International Convention on Psychotropic Substances, signed in Vienna, when Richard Nixon, the man who declared the so-called "war on drugs," was president of the United States.

In the 1980s, another of the world's most famous psychoactive substances, MDMA or ecstasy, came into vogue, being described as a semi-psychedelic and known for its entactogenic-empathogenic effects. It was banned in the United States in 1985 despite an administrative court recommendation to include it in Schedule III controlled substances, given that it is not very toxic and seemed to have psychotherapeutic effects. Despite pressure from some psychiatrists and other mental health professionals who used it for their treatments, the DEA (Drug Enforcement Administration) finally included it in its U.S. Schedule I classification, where the most dangerous substances with no recognized therapeutic value are placed, and in 1985 it was also included in Schedule I of the International Convention on Psychotropic Substances, which lists the most toxic and harmful substances considered to have little or no therapeutic value.

1.2 Criteria for Inclusion in One Control List or Another

Inclusion in one list or another does not always depend so much on the hazardousness or toxicity of the substance, or on its real therapeutic potential, but rather on a political or moral decision influenced by a given spatiotemporal context. In this regard, Nutt, King, and Phillips (2010) established a classification of the dangerousness of different drugs (legal and illegal) using a multitude of criteria, concluding that the least dangerous substances were psychedelic molecules, such as LSD and psilocybin, and semipsychedelics, such as cannabis and MDMA.[3] These substances were placed way below others, such as alcohol and tobacco, which, despite being more harmful, are legal.

In the words of an anonymous administrator and convention participant quoted by Mark Kleiman (professor of public policy and director of the Crime and Justice Program at New York University), ranking decisions are ultimately a consequence of the following premise: "If it's fun, it's Schedule One."[4]

1.3 The International Classification of Ketamine: A Substance with Recognized Medical Uses

The situation is different for ketamine, a substance with psychedelic and dissociative properties that was synthesized in 1962 by Calvin Stevens. Since then it has been used therapeutically in medicine and veterinary

---

3. Nutt DJ, King LA, Phillips LD. 2010. Drug harms in the UK: a multicriteria decision analysis. The Lancet 376(9752):1558–1565.
4. Arbour, et al. 2019. (See full reference in note 2 of this appendix.)

medicine as a general anesthetic and has also been included in the list of essential medicines of the World Health Organization (WHO) by virtue of its usefulness and safety. Since 2019, this substance, or rather one of its purified molecular forms (esketamine), patented by the pharmaceutical company Janssen (owned by Johnson & Johnson), has been

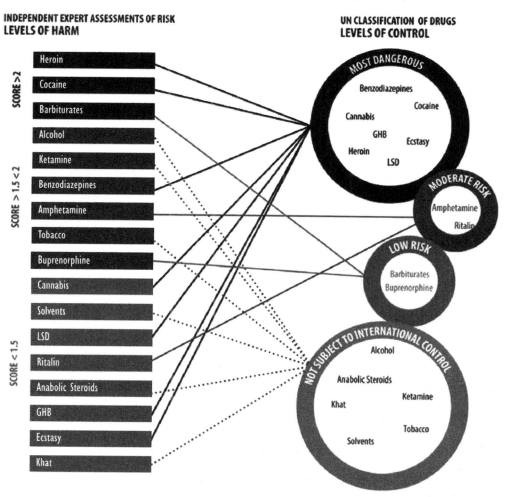

Figure 41. Levels of harm of different drugs as assessed by scientists, compared to their current international legal control levels. Figure adapted from: Nutt D, et al. 2007. Development of a rational scale to assess the harm of drugs of potential misuse. The Lancet 369 No. 9566:1047–53; Gomis B. 2016. Modernising Drug Law Enforcement. International Drug Policy Consortium, Drug Policy Guide, 3rd ed, 90–96.

recognized by the FDA and other drug agencies for the treatment of depression, and, likely, this therapeutic indication will also be extended to racemic (classic) ketamine—though this has not happened yet.

Due to the rise of ketamine for recreational use, it was first controlled in the United States in 1999, and in 2006 it was listed by the United Nations Commission on Narcotic Drugs (CND) as a controlled substance under the 1971 Convention on Psychotropic Substances. Other states then transposed this prohibition into their national laws.

All the substances mentioned up to this point, except ketamine (which is in Schedule IV), are in Schedule I of the 1971 Convention on Psychotropic Substances where (according to the convention) the most dangerous and least valuable drugs in medicine are placed under control. Member states have also included them in the list where the most punishable substances under their respective national penal codes are to be found.

In the case of ketamine, this substance has always been recognized as having therapeutic properties as a general anesthetic and, more recently, as a psychiatric drug for the treatment of severe depression. For this reason, it has always been considered more therapeutic and less dangerous than other drugs; however, this cannot be considered scientifically correct since, for example, according to the report by Nutt et al., 2010, despite being below that of other legal drugs such as alcohol and tobacco, the harmful potential of ketamine for the individual and society is above that of LSD and psilocybin.

The WHO Expert Committee on Drug Dependence acknowledged that some concern had been expressed, stating:

> Placing ketamine under international control would have a negative impact on the availability and accessibility of this substance. This, in turn, would limit access to essential and emergency surgery, leading to a public health crisis in countries where no other affordable replacement anaesthetic is available.[5]

---

5. WHO. 2012. WHO Expert Committee on Drug Dependence, Report No. 35, Technical Report Series 973. Geneva (Switzerland): World Health Organization, 9.

As can be seen, the case of synthetic drugs with psychedelic properties such as ketamine and MDMA or semisynthetic drugs such as LSD
(derived from the ergot fungus) is not technically complicated when
it comes to interpreting their legal status. As we will see below, legal
interpretations become more complicated when dealing with plants or
mushrooms that contain psychotropic controlled molecules.

The historical and legal arguments set out in the introduction to
this appendix require us to navigate the paradoxical legislation and
jurisprudence that regulate this issue.

2. STATES AND CITIES IN THE UNITED STATES THAT HAVE DECRIMINALIZED THE USE OF PSYCHEDELIC SUBSTANCES

2.1 U.S. Cities that Have Pioneered the Decriminalization of Psychedelic Substances

Since 2012, when the states of Colorado and Washington regulated
access to cannabis for recreational use, there have been many efforts by
associations advocating changes in current drug policies. To alleviate the
great pandemic of mental illnesses that is increasingly present in society,
such associations are seeking recognition of their therapeutic uses.

Thus, since then, not only has cannabis been regulated for recreational purposes in more than twenty states and Washington, DC,
there have also been political and legislative movements to decriminalize the use of certain psychedelic substances in many parts of the
United States, both at the state and municipal levels.

The first city to decriminalize the use of a substance other than
cannabis was Denver, Colorado. In 2019, it did not quite legalize
psilocybin (found in magic mushrooms), but it did, however, prohibit
wasting police and judicial efforts to prosecute its use, thus being at
the forefront of decriminalizing psychedelic drugs and recognizing their
therapeutic value.

Other West Coast cities have also joined the reform, such as Oakland,
California (historically very familiar with the use of entheogens), which

in 2019 also decriminalized the use of plants, cacti, and mushrooms containing controlled substances such as psilocybin, mescaline, and DMT; and Santa Cruz, also in California, which in 2020 decriminalized the possession and cultivation of psilocybin-containing magic mushrooms, although the commercial sale of them remains illegal.

Washington, DC, followed suit in November 2020; and in 2021, the cities of Somerville, Bay State, and Cambridge, Massachusetts, did the same. Hence, we are no longer talking exclusively about cities on the West Coast. The decriminalization of psychedelics, like cannabis, has also reached the East Coast.

The latest cities to jump on the psychedelic bandwagon are Seattle (in Washington State), Arcata (in California), and Easthampton (in Massachusetts), which no longer prioritize the prosecution of crimes related to entheogenic plants. It, therefore, seems that, very soon, the possession and use of cannabis and other substances such as psilocybin (magic mushrooms) or mescaline (San Pedro cactus and peyote) will not be prosecuted in most states.

2.2 U.S. States that Have Decriminalized or Legalized the Use of Psychedelics

Regarding the decriminalization of psilocybin at the state level, the state of Oregon was the first to take the big step in November 2020, recognizing its use for therapeutic purposes, as it considers it useful for treating major depression and PTSD. Thus, possession of up to 12 g of magic mushrooms only entails a $100 fine or the completion of a health assessment. The possession of more than 12 g can lead to jail time. What is now completely legal in the state of Oregon is the provision of psilocybin treatments in specialized and certified centers.

The next state that seems to be getting ready to legalize the use of psilocybin for medicinal purposes is the state of California, where several proposals to legalize magic mushrooms' psychoactive molecule and other entheogenic plants for medicinal purposes have already been put forward. As of this writing, there are also such proposals in the states of New York and New Jersey.

2.3 Potential Problems Where U.S. Federal Law Comes into Play

Although these reforms are taking place at the local and state level, the United States is a federal republic, and U.S. federal law still includes psilocybin in its Schedule I controlled substances, which are considered the most dangerous and have the fewest therapeutic uses. This means that, even if they are in a city or state that has already decriminalized them if a person is caught in possession of these substances by FBI agents, they can be charged with possession of illegal drugs under U.S. federal law.

2.4 Conclusion

In summary, since some American cities don't consider them to be harmful and do instead consider them to have increasingly recognized therapeutic value, they are no longer prioritizing the efforts of their local police to prosecute people who use this type of drug. However, the only state that has legalized psilocybin for medicinal purposes is Oregon, and the U.S. Congress, which legislates at the federal level on drug issues, is not yet in favor of legalizing such substances. Therefore, the reader of this book should take special care if in possession of a certain quantity of substances considered psychedelic, as, with a few local exceptions, they are still prohibited nationally and, of course, internationally in all countries.

3. GRADUATION OF PENALTIES FOR TRAFFICKING AND USE OF PSYCHEDELIC SUBSTANCES AROUND THE WORLD

In order to impose a penalty on the offender, drug trafficking offenses in countries that follow the rule of law are usually classified based on three basic factors: the alleged dangerousness of the substance, the quantity seized, and the aggravating circumstances of the case.

3.1 Increased Penalties for the Dangerousness of the Substance

In order to assess the criminal risks that would exist in cases of arrest for possession or sale of these substances, it should first be checked whether or not the member state in question is signed on to the 1971 United Nations Convention, whether or not it has also transposed the convention into national law (i.e., whether such signed international convention has been "translated" into national law), and finally, whether those particular substances are controlled in any of the schedules of the national drug law of each state.

> Despite this, there are countries with analogue laws: the US Analogue Substances Act, enacted in 1988, which automatically bans a substance if its structure and effects are "substantially similar" to those of an already banned drug; or the UK's Psychoactive Substances Act of 2016, which by default bans any psychoactive substance that by stimulating or depressing the person's central nervous system . . . affects the person's mental functioning or emotional state.[6]

Penalties are usually imposed according to whether substances are more or less dangerous to public health. Some countries such as the United Kingdom classify them in Schedules A, B, or C, with the most (officially) dangerous substances such as cocaine, heroin, LSD, and psilocybin placed in Schedule A, amphetamines and cannabis in Schedule B, and tranquilizers in Schedule C. The United States also has five schedules, included in the first schedule those substances that are allegedly most abused, most toxic, and not medically licensed (LSD, psilocybin, DMT, and 2CB), with ketamine, for example, being included in Schedule III, given it is medically licensed.

The case of Spain, for example, is more complex, having transposed the international drug conventions into domestic law by copying the same substances included in the schedules of the aforementioned international convention. Therefore, in the case of psychotropics, substances in Schedule I are officially more dangerous, and with less recognized therapeutic value, than those in Schedules II, III, and IV.

---

6. United Kingdom. 2016. Psychoactive Substances Act. London: Crown, paragraph 2. Retrieved from the U.K. government website.

However, Article 36[7] of the Spanish Penal Code establishes a penal difference depending on whether or not the substance can cause serious damage to health. Paradoxically, however, this concept is not normative (not defined in the law), but jurisprudential (applied based on what previous judgments have interpreted), because the only drug currently classified by the jurisprudence of the Spanish courts as not causing serious harm to health is cannabis, and it is in Schedule I (the most controlled and with the least therapeutic potential) of the Spanish Narcotics Law 17/1967, while amphetamines and 2CB are in Schedule II (less controlled), although they are treated by case law as causing serious harm to health—yet another case of nonsensical legislation.

It should be noted that this jurisprudential concept, that of serious damage to health, is subject to change through the provision of pharmacological expert evidence, that is, what experts on the substance can say in court about its dangerousness. In fact, for example, MDMA (ecstasy) was considered by the Spanish National Court as a substance that does not cause serious damage to health in a hearing in 1994 in which the expert witness for the defense was Alexander Shulgin himself, considered the godfather or rediscoverer of this substance, as well as the mastermind behind the expansion of its use among the therapeutic community to treat post-traumatic stress disorder and other psychiatric illnesses. During the trial, the scientist compared MDMA to its chemical "big sister," MDA, to explain that MDMA is less neurotoxic than MDA and that it does not have high addictive power. Thanks to testimony, the court decided to consider ecstasy a substance that does not cause serious damage to health (Yoldi 1994) and was therefore made punishable by a lesser penalty than cocaine and LSD. However, later on, Spanish court jurisprudence changed its opinion, considering ecstasy (MDMA) a health hazard. This was possibly due to the Leah Betts scandal, the eighteen-year-old British girl who died after taking an

7. Yoldi J. 1994 Jan 23. El éxtasis no causa grave daño a la salud según la Audiencia Nacional [Ecstasy does not cause serious health effects, according to the National Court of Spain]. El País (Madrid). Spanish.

ecstasy pill at a house party with her parents. During the days when she was in a coma, a media campaign made the front page of newspapers in the United Kingdom and around the world, publishing photos of her on her deathbed and filling the streets up with pictures of her face accompanied by messages about the dangers of drugs. Later, the doctor who treated her said that she had died from overhydration, known as hyponatremia, as she drank too much water in an attempt to quash the effect of the pill. In reality, deaths from ecstasy use are not common and occur much less frequently than those related to alcohol or tobacco,[8] without resulting in the criminalization of their possession or distribution.

3.2 Increasing Penalties for Quantity Seized

The different countries that have banned the possession and sale of different psychedelic (or other) drugs also tend to establish tables to increase penalties according to the quantity of the substance seized.

This is the case, for example, in the United States, which has tables of equivalence between substances in which, if a certain quantity is exceeded, the minimum or maximum penalty required by federal law is increased. In the case of ecstasy, for example, there is a table of equivalence concerning cannabis, with the equivalence being 1–500. This means that 1 g of MDMA is equivalent to the penalty for 500 g of cannabis. This equivalence was raised in 2001 from 35–1 to 500–1, but in 2011, with the collaboration of the Multidisciplinary Association for Psychedelic Studies (MAPS), it was set by two American courts at 200–1, considering that the scientific reports provided in 2001 were based on exaggerated, and scientifically unsound, perceptions of the harmfulness of MDMA, and that MDMA was no more harmful than cocaine. In 2017, an attempt was made to reclassify the equivalence of ecstasy in a proceeding in which Dr. Rick Doblin, the founder of MAPS, was an expert witness, without succeeding in having the

8. Collin M. 2002. Estado alterado: la historia de la cultura del éxtasis y del acid house [Altered state: the history of ecstasy culture and "acid house"]. Barcelona (Spain): Alba Editorial. Spanish.

dangerousness of MDMA reconsidered.[9] However, with the work of people like Doblin and MAPS, MDMA is now in phase 3 clinical trials, and FDA recognition for the treatment of post-traumatic stress disorder and other psychiatric illnesses is expected by 2024.

3.3 Increased Penalties for Aggravating Circumstances

Penalties are also often increased for other aggravating circumstances, such as committing a crime with violence, belonging to a criminal organization, or trafficking minors.

Sentences for drug trafficking are typically set at between two and ten years in most countries, rising to twenty years or even life imprisonment in countries such as the United States or the United Kingdom, when there are very special and specific circumstances such as the use of criminal gangs or violence. There are regions where sentences can be particularly high, such as Africa, the Middle East, and Asia.

3.4 Tolerance in Cases of Small Quantities for Personal Use

In most European countries, some U.S. states, Canada, and in most South American countries, drug use for personal use is tolerated, and offenses for simple possession of drugs are usually punishable by a prison sentence of between six months and two years, which may be suspended if the offender is a first offender (no previous criminal record) or undergoing drug detoxification treatment. It might also just be replaced by a fine.[10]

However, the specific legislation in each country needs to be studied in detail to find out whether there is a law for minimum dose for

---

9. Multidisciplinary Association for Psychedelic Studies USSC Testimony re: MDMA March 15, 2017.

10. Cavada JP. 2020. Criterios para el sancionamiento del consumo o tráfico de drogas en el derecho extranjero [Criteria for the punishment of drug use or trafficking abroad]. Santiago de Chile: Biblioteca Nacional del Congreso de Chile. Spanish. Retrieved from the Biblioteca Nacional del Congreso de Chile website.

personal use or whether simple possession is punishable by administrative fines and the like.

3.4.1 Latin American Countries

Latin American countries such as Colombia, Uruguay, Peru, and Mexico have minimum personal dose laws, in which small quantities of various substances cannot even be punished by an administrative rule.

In Peru, for example, drug trafficking is punishable by a sentence of eight to fifteen years, and possession for the purpose of trafficking is punishable by six to twelve years, and even life imprisonment if forced by violence or intimidation to plant drugs. However, possession for the personal use of up to 5 g of cocaine base paste, 2 g of cocaine hydrochloride, 8 g of marijuana, and 2 g of its derivatives, or 250 milligrams of MDMA or similar substances[11] is not criminalized. Having said this, it seems that the dose is seized even if it is not sanctioned in all countries except Uruguay.[12]

In Mexico and Colombia, for example, the constitutional courts have issued two rulings, on November 4, 2015, and June 6, 2019, respectively, in which, in the section on the weighing of affected fundamental rights and collective legal interests to be protected (public health and safety), it is concluded that these two collective interests should not prevail over the individual freedom and free development of the personality of the drug user, as long as the test of proportionality in the interpretation of these affected fundamental rights and protected legal interests is not passed. In other words, individual liberties prevail over the personal consumption of substances in the face of other considerations, such as public health and safety, allegedly threatened by personal drug consumption. However, the Colombian Constitutional Court had

---

11. Martín A, Muñoz J. 2019. El estatuto legal de la ayahuasca en España: la relevancia penal de los comportamientos relacionados con su consumo y posesión [Legal status of ayahuasca in Spain: the criminal relevance of behaviors related to its consumption and possession]. Valencia (Spain): Tirant lo Blanch. Spanish.
12. Salvo Uruguay, dosis mínima se incauta en toda A. Latina [With the exception of Uruguay, minimum doses are seized throughout Latin America]. El Nuevo Siglo (Bogotá, Colombia) 2018 Sept 6. Spanish.

already declared the criminalization of drug use unconstitutional in Ruling C-221/94. Despite this ruling almost two decades ago, subsequent governments have criticized this judicial decision and attempted to recriminalize drug use for personal consumption, generating laws that currently prohibit use but do not criminalize it. This ruling was used by academic researchers and by countries such as Switzerland and the Netherlands to adapt their arguments for their legislation.[13]

In Argentina, penalties range from one month to two years imprisonment, plus a fine for possession for personal use (Art. 14, second paragraph, Law 23.737); from one to six years imprisonment, plus a fine for simple possession (first paragraph of the same article); and from four to fifteen years imprisonment, plus a fine for possession for commercial purposes (5 inc. C of the same law). The latter Article 5 also establishes penalties for trafficking of four to fifteen years imprisonment, plus a fine, and some aggravating circumstances are described in subsequent articles. Cross-border trafficking is punishable under the Customs Code (Art. 866), with penalties ranging from four and a half months to sixteen years.

3.4.2 The Spanish Case

In Spain, as long as no specific quantities of psychedelics are found that exceed what is considered usual for daily personal use for three to five days, and provided there are no indications of trafficking (such as having the substance divided into doses, having a precision scale, a multitude of substances, a notebook with notes, cash, and so on), the case would not be sent to a criminal court. This has been established by the National Institute of Toxicology at a maximum of 2.4 g of pure MDMA or 0.003 g of LSD,[14] with a fine of between 601 and 30,000 euros[15] being imposed in these cases. However, this law is to

---

13. Uprimny R. 2019. A 25 años de la sentencia C-221/94 en Colombia: una oportunidad perdida [Twenty-five years after the C-221/94 sentence in Colombia: a missed opportunity]. London: International Drug Policy Consortium. Spanish. Retrieved from the International Drug Policy Consortium website.
14. Instituto Nacional de Toxicología (2001). Informe sobre dosis mínima psicoactiva, de 18 de octubre de 2001 [Report on minimum psychoactive dose, October 18, 2001]. Madrid: Instituto Nacional de Toxicología. Spanish.

be amended shortly, and it seems that fines for simple possession will be considered minor (the amount would be between 100 and 600 euros), and consumption on public roads will be punished with a fine of 601 euros.[16] However, perhaps because they are less prevalent in the population, substances such as psilocybin are not included in this table of quantities regarding personal consumption, nor do they appear in tables in other countries. In this case, and in order to calculate the dose that could be regarded as for personal use, and what quantities could be considered as trafficking and therefore subject to higher penalties, ad hoc expert evidence will be required. Despite exceeding the National Institute of Toxicology (INT) quantities, Spanish jurisprudence requires proof of intent to traffic the substance to convict through other evidence or indications.

To further highlight the lack of solid scientific criteria when establishing penalties for drug trafficking in Spain, we can recover this excerpt from an article on the words spoken by the director of INT at the time of issuing the famous report:

> "That table was part of a technical report that was sent in 2001 to the Supreme Court, but at no point did we address whether they should be used to set sentences or not," Gómez explained. Gómez agreed with the opinions of other experts consulted, and clarified that "the effect of a toxic substance on the organism depends on the person, their size, their state and how used to it they are. It is the same as with Valium which doesn't have the same effect on everyone. Some people fall asleep with one pill, others don't feel anything when they take two."[17]

---

15. Ley Orgánica 4/2015, de 30 de marzo, de protección de la seguridad ciudadana [Organic Law 4/2015, March 30, on the protection of public safety]. Published in BOE [Official State Bulletin] No. 77, March 31, 2015. Spanish.

16. Azorín F. 2021 Dec 14. Reforma de la Ley Mordaza y cannabis: es urgente [Reform of the "Gag Rule" and cannabis: it's urgent]. El Salto (Madrid). Spanish.

17. Lázaro JM, De Benito E. 2004 Apr 11. Toxicología se desmarca del baremo que utiliza el Supremo para condenar a 'camellos' [Toxicology disassociates itself from the scale used by the Supreme Court to sentence "dealers"]. El País (Madrid). Spanish.

In other words, not even the authors of the report considered it fair that sentences should be passed based on this technical report. As historically only a summary table has been available on the internet, I requested the report via Spain's Transparency Portal. It came as a great surprise to see that there were no bibliographical references that could be refuted by other experts through contradictory expert evidence. Only a legend full of scientific and logical deficiencies could be found. For example, all substances have a range of daily doses, and to obtain the maximum amount for personal use, the highest end of the range is multiplied by 5 (in reference to five days of personal use). However, in the case of MDMA (ecstasy), it is stated that between one and fifteen tablets of 80 mg can be consumed per day when, according to the report, the norm is to take six tablets per day (which goes against the logic of the table, which always multiplies by 5 the highest dose of the range).

3.4.3 Personal Use Doses for Non-Scheduled Substances

In those cases where the substance in question does not appear in the table, it is up to the police to decide whether, depending on the dose seized, a case should be dealt with under criminal or administrative law. However, as we have said, the tables are not complete and do not cover the full range of psychopharmacological drugs used by people who consume illegal substances. In fact, in the case of psilocybin mushrooms, there is an acquittal in Spain that states the following:

In the specific case of the ruling, 670 mushrooms weighing 202.5 grams were seized. In this sense, the minimum active dose [of pure psilocybin] is around 2 milligrams, 10 to 20 milligrams is a medium dose, and a high dose is 30 milligrams or more. The effects of medium doses last for 4 to 6 hours and those of high doses for up to 8 hours. Based on these parameters, the daily dose of [pure psilocybin] consumption can be put at around 100 mg. If we multiply this amount by 1.7 mg of psilocybin per mushroom, the result is just

over 1 gram of this substance [pure psilocybin]. This is an amount
that guarantees consumption for about 10 days.[18]

The reader will note, if experienced in the use of mushrooms, that,
when it comes to psychedelics such as mushrooms or LSD, which are
usually taken very infrequently, in annual or monthly doses at most,
this ruling does not make much sense. However, drug jurisprudence is
often constructed by people with little knowledge of the subject who
assume that everyone who takes drugs is addicted and that taking a
substance necessarily implies continuous use throughout the day to be
under its effects twenty-four hours a day, every day. This flawed logic
is probably derived from the problematic use of certain highly addictive
opiates, such as heroin.

3.4.4 The Dutch Case
In the Netherlands, for example, possession of up to 5 g of fresh mushrooms and 0.5 g of dried mushrooms used to be tolerated, but in 2008,
fresh mushrooms were explicitly banned. Previously, only dried mushrooms were considered to be "a preparation containing psilocybin" as
defined by the 1971 Psychotropic Convention. Since 2008, the market
switched from mushrooms to psilocybin-containing truffles, given that
these fungal species were not explicitly controlled.[19]

3.4.5 Portugal and Its Risk and Harm Reduction Policy
Another country where possession of drugs for personal use is not
criminalized is Portugal. Law 30/2000, adopted in November 2000
and enforced since July 2001, decriminalized the consumption,
acquisition, and possession of drugs for personal use. A decree establishes the quantities that will not lead to criminal prosecution for
each substance, estimating as a maximum the daily consumption of
a drug for a period of ten days. If someone is caught consuming in

---

18. Sentence from the Audiencia Provincial of Alicante No. 129/2013 February 28.
19. Legal situation of psilocybin mushrooms. Obtained from Wikipedia.

the street, they are given the option of attending an interview with a committee comprised of a psychologist, a social worker, and a jurist so that they can analyze whether the situation is considered problematic consumption and, if so, offer the consumer therapeutic help (Cavada 2020).

3.4.6 France and Italy and Their Hardline Drug Policy

France, for its part, has always been a very belligerent country on drug issues within Europe. However, penalties for simple possession are less than one year, plus a fine, and the offender is usually required to attend and pay for a drug awareness course (Cavada 2020).

Italy is another country that establishes higher penalties for drug trafficking offenses, especially if committed by organized mafias. In terms of penalties for simple possession, it is also a rather tough country because, even if criminal proceedings are not initiated, serious administrative sanctions, such as the loss of one's driver's license, could be imposed. The country also offers substitution treatments for confiscations where no evidence of drug trafficking exists.[20]

3.4.7 Other European Countries

Concerning the tables of doses for personal use in other European countries, the European Monitoring Centre for Drugs and Drug Addiction (EMCDDA) produces summary tables for each country, available in the "Publications" section of the EMCDDA website ("Threshold quantities for drug offences").

3.5 *Conclusion*

In conclusion, in most countries that have a legal system based on the rule of law, with constitutions that protect and recognize fundamental rights of the individual, simple possession of drugs for personal use is not usually punishable by imprisonment. And if a prison term for personal use is stated in the law, it is usually symbolic and

---

20. Cavada JP. 2020. (See full reference in note 10 of this appendix.)

probably will be suspended if the person is a first offender or undergoes drug treatment. However, each factual situation can be interpreted in different ways, depending on the case, so to minimize the legal risks of possession and use, the drug user should do his or her part to understand how the supposed tolerance of personal possession for the personal use of drugs is interpreted in the legal practice of the relevant country.

3.6 Special Caution in Countries with Strict Drug Laws

In some countries around the world, especially in Africa, the Middle East, and Asia, what we in the West would call a "rule of law with due process and recognition of individual rights" is not strictly enforced. Therefore, drug possession in countries such as the Philippines, China, India, Malaysia, Qatar, Saudi Arabia, and others can lead to very serious problems with the law. Paradoxically, it seems that Thailand,[21] one of these countries, intends to regulate recreational cannabis soon, having regulated access to the plant for medicinal purposes in 2020. It seems that drug policy is changing dramatically in some countries, and not necessarily only in Western ones or those with a democratic culture that, through the rule of law, recognizes the individual's fundamental rights.

4. INTERNATIONAL CONTROL OF PLANTS CONTAINING MOLECULES CLASSIFIED AS PSYCHOTROPIC UNDER THE 1971 CONVENTION

As mentioned above, when we encounter interceptions of plant or fungal substances containing a molecule classified as psychotropic under the 1971 Convention on Psychotropic Substances, the legal interpretation becomes quite complicated.

---

21. Tailandia, primer país de Asia que despenaliza la marihuana [Thailand, the first country to decriminalize marijuana]. Diario Las Américas (Miami, FL) 2022 Jan 25. Spanish.

4.1 The International Narcotics Control Board's Interpretation of the Conventions

In this section, we will analyze the thesis of the International Narcotics Control Board (INCB) when applying the international conventions to certain psychoactive plants that are not expressly controlled but contain substances that are.

The INCB or NCBI, in its 2010 and 2012 reports, states that there are only three plants controlled by the international drug conventions. These are only the cannabis plant (*C. sativa*); the coca leaf (*Erythroxylum coca*), from which cocaine is extracted; and the white poppy (*Papaver somniferum*), from which the opium needed to make morphine and heroin is extracted. In other words, the 1961 Convention on Narcotic Drugs only banned certain plants.

Although some active ingredients with stimulant or hallucinogenic effects contained in certain plants are controlled under the 1971 Convention, no plants are currently controlled under that convention or the 1988 Convention. Nor are preparations (e.g., decoctions for oral consumption) made from plants containing such active ingredients under international control.

Examples of such plants or plant materials are khat (*Catha edulis*), whose active ingredients cathinone and cathine are included in Schedules I and III of the 1971 Convention; ayahuasca, originating in the Amazon basin, mainly consisting of a preparation of *Banisteriopsis caapi* (a jungle vine) and another tryptamine-rich plant (*P. viridis*) that contains various psychoactive alkaloids such as DMT.[22]

No plants, even those containing psychoactive ingredients, are currently controlled under the 1971 Convention, although in some cases the active ingredients they contain may be under international control. For example, cathine and DMT are psychotropic substances listed in Schedule I of the 1971 Convention, while the plants and herbal preparations containing them, namely khat and

---

22. International Narcotics Control Board. 2011. 2010 Report. United Nations. New York.

ayahuasca, respectively, are not subject to any restriction or control measures.[23]

4.2 Possibility of Some Countries Controlling Certain Psychoactive Plants on an Individual Basis

Despite the explanation in the previous section, there may be countries that have expressly prohibited plants or parts of plants, as is the case in France with ayahuasca and in the Netherlands with magic mushrooms.

However, despite the interpretations of the International Narcotics Control Board, the truth is that, in most countries, seizures of ayahuasca are indeed reported and the police do usually confiscate magic mushrooms.

In Spain, most of the judicial precedents of criminal courts and provincial courts have considered that ayahuasca is not subject to the control regime of international treaties and that, therefore, its possession or sale is not criminally relevant.

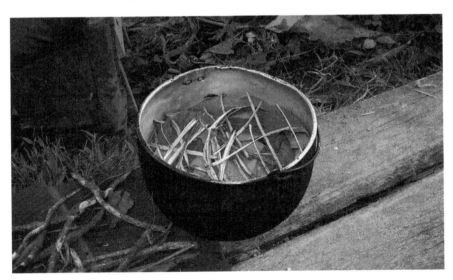

Figure 42. Ayahuasca, ready to be cooked. Terpsichore, CC BY-SA 3.0, via Wikimedia Commons.

23. International Narcotics Control Board. 2013. 2012 Report. United Nations. New York.

Thus, one of the latest court rulings, obtained by Francisco Azorín Ortega, the author of this appendix, states:

> To recapitulate, at the international level it seems clear that, either in its plant presentation or as a preparation (paradigmatically decoction for oral ingestion, which is the case here), ayahuasca cannot be understood to be included in the 1971 Convention, even though DMT is; and therefore, as a decoction or in its plant presentation (the plants from which it is obtained), it is not subject to international control.
>
> As a conclusion of this absence of specific mention at the national level and the lack of legal coverage in the 1971 Convention for its inclusion, we, therefore, understand that this preparation is not subject to special control in Spain, nor can it, therefore, be included in the definition of Article 368 of the Criminal Code.[24]

4.3 Pre-Trial Detention for False Positive Methamphetamine Tests

A person who was eventually acquitted for receiving a package with ayahuasca from Peru spent three months in prison because the substance showed a false positive for methamphetamine in the presumptive colorimetric test carried out by the police (something that usually happens with these plants). Therefore, until the substance was analyzed by a laboratory, with a confirmatory test, and until the corresponding appeals were filed because ayahuasca is not controlled, the investigated prisoner could not be released. Despite this, the antidrug prosecutor's office charged him with a crime against public health and asked for four years in prison.

There are also cases in which the investigating courts have ordered provisional imprisonment for the seizure of tobacco snuffs called rapé, sometimes containing DMT, which can show a false positive result for

---

24. Sentence from the Provincial Court (Audiencia Provincial) of Málaga (Sección 1ª) No. 86/2021 March 10.

amphetamine or MDMA in the presumptive colorimetric tests carried out at customs. Even though a document from the Spanish Customs and Excise Department states that—even though almost all proceedings end in a file or acquittal and, normally, people who travel with suitcases loaded with ayahuasca from Colombia or Peru are no longer sent to provisional prison—controlled deliveries of ayahuasca should not be carried out, the truth is that as the appearance of these is that of a substance in greyish powder form that gives a false positive for MDMA, there have been provisional incarcerations for such rapés. In other words, if 3 or 4 kilos of rapés are seized and thus produce a false positive result, it is easy to be sent to prison until the health department determines, in a confirmatory manner, the substance in question and its quantification, an injustice that confirms the deficiencies of the system and the lack of public resources and knowledge when it comes to the state exercising its greatest power, the punitive power, or what the Romans called *ultima ratio* or the ultimate "reason of state": criminal law. Pretrial detentions have been criticized multiple times by the renowned criminal justice lawyer Gerardo Landrove Díaz as "legalized injustice."

5. COUNTRIES THAT HAVE RECOGNIZED OR BANNED CERTAIN PLANTS WITH CONTROLLED MOLECULES AS PSYCHOTROPIC

5.1 Lack of Clarity in the Wording of International Conventions

As mentioned above, the legal interpretation of the international accounting of plants containing molecules controlled as psychotropic by the 1971 Convention has never been simple or peaceful and has always generated controversy.

All this controversy stems from the wording of the international conventions and their official commentaries.

Sánchez and Bouso (2015) state in a report:

What does not seem to be so clear is whether, in order to continue allowing the traditional use of these psychoactive plants, a state party to the convention must formulate a reservation or not. Reading the text of the treaty, one would say yes. But the commentary introduces a statement that, in a way, creates a paradox concerning what the convention itself establishes: when it says that "... Continued tolerance of the use of the hallucinogenic substances mentioned at the 1971 Conference does not require the formulation of a reservation under paragraph 4 of Article 32 since, following the traditional way of dealing with this issue in the framework of international drug control, the commentators consider that 'the inclusion in Schedule I of the active ingredient of a substance does not mean that the substance itself is also included in the Schedule if it is a substance clearly distinct from the substance which constitutes its active ingredient.'"

Therefore, there exists a disparity between the text of the convention and its official commentary signed by the U.N. Secretary-General. This discrepancy was clarified by the INCB in the above-mentioned reports of 2010 and 2012, which stated that these plants are not subject to international control.[25]

5.2 Countries that Have Made Exceptions to International Conventions and Rulings Clarifying This Issue

Only Mexico, Peru, the United States, and Canada have indeed made reservations to the 1971 international treaty to allow certain traditional uses of these substances by native communities in the Amazon basin or Indigenous reservations in the United States and Canada.[26]

In Chile, for example, a judgment was handed down in 2012

---

25. Sánchez C, Bouso JC. 2015. Ayahuasca: de la Amazonía a la aldea global [Ayahuasca: from the Amazon to the global village]. Barcelona (Spain): International Center for Ethnobotanical Education, Research, and Service. Spanish. Retrieved from the Transnational Institute website.
26. Sánchez C, Bouso JC. 2015. (See full reference in note 25 of this appendix.)

(Manto Wasi case) in which an ayahuasca ceremony had been infiltrated by a police officer. It was considered that ayahuasca could not be identified with DMT, controlled by the 1971 international convention and Decree No. 867 of 2007 of the Andean country controlling DMT, but that *P. viridis* and *B. cappi*, the individual plant components used to prepare ayahuasca, could be. The ruling stated that ayahuasca did not pose a danger to public health, and following the case, the director of public health requested that the Ministry of the Interior control ayahuasca. The initiative did not go forward.[27]

France, however, does follow a prohibitionist model. In 1999, a controversy arose over a complaint by a mother of a member of a daimist group[28] who claimed that her son had lost touch with reality. The case resulted in a conviction by the Paris Court of First Instance on January 15, 2004. The ruling was appealed to the Paris Court of Appeal, which ruled on January 13, 2015, that, although ayahuasca has hallucinogenic effects, it can be distinguished from synthetic DMT, which is what is undoubtedly subject to the prohibition under French law. Furthermore, it was not possible to speak of a preparation in the technical and legal sense, as this would require the existence of a pure substance. As a result, the court ruled in favor of acquittal (Martín and Muñoz 2019). This pronouncement caused alarm among the authorities who, in order to avoid the situation highlighted in the ruling, decided to include all plants that are used or usually used in ayahuasca decoctions in the decree of April 20, 2005, thus prohibiting the uses of this plant in France (Martín and Muñoz 2019).

---

27. Martín A, Muñoz J. 2019. (See full reference in note 11 of this appendix.)

28. Santo Daime is a syncretic spiritual practice that blends elements of Christianity with South American Indigenous traditions and African influences. Originating in the Brazilian Amazon in the 1930s, it was founded by Raimundo Irineu Serra, known as Mestre Irineu. Central to the Santo Daime religion is the sacramental consumption of ayahuasca, a psychoactive brew traditionally used by Indigenous peoples for spiritual and healing purposes.

5.3 Religious Uses and Cultural Heritage

In Brazil, a country with a strong "ayahuasca" culture, religious uses are recognized. Moreover, Brazil has not made a reservation to the 1971 Convention, and in 1985 the Ministry of Health included *B. cappi* and *P. viridis* as controlled substances. However, the "ayahuasca church," the União do Vegetal (UDV), fought a legal battle, which led to a study being carried out in communities that use ayahuasca in order to show that it had a significant positive effect (absence of alcoholism, lower infant mortality and malnutrition, crime rates close to zero, absence of violence, and the like). As a result of this report, the exclusion of plant species used in the preparation of ayahuasca was declared by Resolution No. 6 of February 4, 1986 (Martín and Muñoz 2019).

Subsequently, Resolution No. 1 of May 25, 2010, of CONAD (Council on Narcotic Drugs) ratified the legitimacy of the religious use of ayahuasca in one of the most detailed documents to date, regulating the uses of ayahuasca in religious practices, prohibiting its commercialization for profit, and emphasizing the avoidance of the offering in tourist packages (Martín and Muñoz 2019).

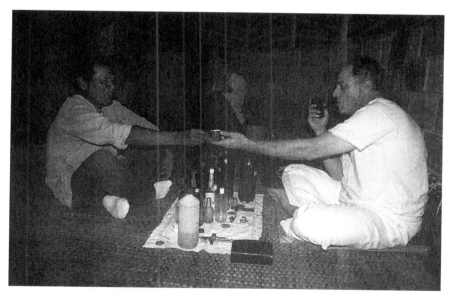

Figure 43. Ayahuasca ceremony at the Takiwasi Center (Peru).
Image by Takiwasi.

Peru, for its part, was the only country to make a distinction, under Article 32 of the 1971 Convention, regarding plants containing Schedule I psychotropic substances that have been traditionally used by certain small, clearly defined groups in religious ceremonies. This happened in 2008 when it declared ayahuasca a national cultural heritage. However, in contrast to Brazil, there is no detailed regulation, but rather a set of customs and practices.

Canada, the United States, and Colombia also allow religious uses of ayahuasca, and Canada and the United States also allow peyote cacti. In the Netherlands, religious uses of ayahuasca were allowed, but a Supreme Court ruling in 2019 changed the criteria and considered that the right to health prevails over religious freedom, declaring such use illegal.[29]

5.4 Attempts to Ban a Multitude of Medicinal Plants by the Spanish State

In 2004, an attempt was made in Spain to ban by ministerial order a list of 197 plants that were considered toxic or dangerous by the government at the time. The case was appealed before the Audiencia Nacional, which, as well as the Supreme Court in its ruling of July 9, 2008, nullified the ministerial order of January 28, 2004, on the grounds of formal errors in the order. The prohibition of these plants was not attempted again in Spain, so they are not subject to national control, or, as we saw earlier, to international control.

5.5 The Case of Peyote: Countries that Made Exceptions and Those that Consider It Illegal

Regarding peyote, a report by the ICEERS Foundation states: "There are more than forty North American Indian tribes in many parts of the United States and Canada that use peyote as a religious sacrament."

The psychoactive alkaloid in peyote, mescaline, is a controlled sub-

---

29. Ferrer I. 2019 Oct 2. El Supremo holandés prohíbe la importación de ayahuasca [Dutch Supreme Court bans the importation of ayahuasca]. El País (Madrid). Spanish.

stance under the 1971 Vienna Convention and is included in Schedule I. Its use, sale, and manufacture are therefore prohibited. However, the peyote plant is not included in the schedules of the conventions, and its regulation depends on the legislation of each country. Thus, in Canada, mescaline is in Schedule III, and peyote is explicitly exempted from regulation if it is not prepared for ingestion, whereas in Brazil, France, Italy, and other countries, peyote is considered illegal. Other countries, such as Spain, do not mention peyote in the lists of controlled plants, although this does not imply that the sale of peyote cannot be considered an illegal act.

In the case of U.S. legislation, the use of peyote is permitted only in ceremonial contexts for persons belonging to the Native American Church.

The Mexican government was one of the countries that, when adhering to the 1971 Convention and ratifying it on 20 February 1975, made an express reservation about its application, as there are certain Indigenous ethnic groups on its territory that traditionally use wild plants containing Schedule I psychotropic substances, including peyote. Within Mexican legislation, peyote cactus is not properly prohibited or regulated, as it is not included in any section of the General Health Law. Its use is permitted to the Huichols. Even so, peyote is considered an endangered plant, so, with exception of traditional use by Indigenous peoples, its collection is prohibited.[30]

6. DIFFERENCES BETWEEN CRIMINAL SIGNIFICANCE AND ADMINISTRATIVE REGULATION OF PLANTS CONTAINING MOLECULES CLASSIFIED AS PSYCHOTROPIC

To be fully aware of the legality surrounding these substances, it is necessary to differentiate between criminal and administrative legality. The

---

30. Peyote: basic information. Retrieved from the ICEERS website.

truth is that the uses of ayahuasca and other plants are not authorized at the administrative level in almost any country in the world. Only certain religious uses exist, as we have pointed out in the previous section. In other words, plants with controlled substances cannot be sold as food or medicine, even if they are not expressly prohibited by international conventions or national laws transposing these conventions into national law.

6.1 Projections for Recognition of Medical Use of Psychedelics in the Short Term

This lack of administrative recognition will be short-lived. Clinical trials with psilocybin, MDMA, LSD, ibogaine, and DMT are well advanced, and it is expected that the use of these substances will soon be authorized by the U.S., Canadian, European, and worldwide drug agencies for the treatment of depression, PTSD, anxiety, addictions, and other medical conditions.

6.2 The Canadian Case

Even though they are controlled, due to scientific advances in the recognition of the therapeutic properties of these molecules, their advanced clinical research stage into phases 2 and 3, the safety shown so far, and the need for new drugs in this field, given the delicate mental health situation exacerbated by the pandemic, the Canadian Health Agency (Health Canada) has just authorized doctors' access to psychedelic substances for mental health treatment.

In practice, this means that, in cases where other therapies have failed, are inadequate, or are unavailable in Canada, physicians are able, on behalf of patients with serious or life-threatening conditions, to apply for access to restricted medicines through Canada's Health Special Access Program (SAP).[31]

The proposed amendments are not intended to promote or encourage the early use of unapproved drugs, nor to circumvent well-established

---

31. Canada Gazette, Part I, Volume 154, No. 50: Government Notices. 2020 Dec 12.

clinical trial or drug review and approval processes. However, these amendments could provide an additional potential option for physicians treating patients with serious or life-threatening conditions where other therapies have failed, are not suitable, or are not available.

As mentioned above, for the time being, ketamine or its isolate, esketamine, is the only substance that is currently fully administratively recognized. But very soon there will be more. Not only will cannabis be an administratively recognized medicine, but other, no less important substances (MDMA, psilocybin, DMT, and the like) are also knocking on the door to have their therapeutic properties recognized. One can already hear them: knock, knock!

In conclusion, the past and present research driven by people like Alexander Shulgin, Rick Doblin, Claudio Naranjo, David Nutt, Jordi Riba, Roland Griffiths, Amanda Fielding, José Carlos Bouso, Robin Carhart-Harris, the author of this book, and many others, will soon allow new substances, substances that have been unjustly stigmatized, demonized, abandoned, and banned for more than sixty years, to be authorized in order to deal more effectively with the pandemic of mental illness that plagues our societies.

7. HISTORICAL, ECOLOGICAL, AND CULTURAL REASONS WHY PLANTS WITH MOLECULES CLASSIFIED AS PSYCHOTROPIC WERE NOT BANNED

7.1 Historical and Cultural Reasons

The historical, ecological, and cultural reasons for this choice are varied, but we could say that plants containing the alkaloid dimethyltryptamine (DMT) and mushrooms containing psilocybin are very numerous and are found all over the world. This means that legislators would have to control substances that could grow naturally in any field or garden patch.

One of the most important books ever written on psychedelics, *TiHKAL*, authored by two of the world's most influential people in the study of psychedelics, Alexander and Ann Shulgin,[32] contains a chapter titled "DMT Is Everywhere."

The chapter "Botany of Tryptamines" can be found within the third part of the book and at its beginning, we can read the following:

> What is at the top of the pyramid? N,N-dimethyltryptamine, or DMT, of course. I think this is the right time to talk about the substance and the Drug Law, as 1966 is an interesting time when both stories converge. Manske first synthesised DMT in 1931. It was then independently isolated from two different plants: in 1946 by Goncalves de Lima (from *Mimosa hostilis*) and in 1955 by Fish, Johnson, and Horning (from *Piptadenia peregrina*). In 1956 Szára reported its activity in humans as a synthetic entity. The first legal restrictions on its research came in 1966 in response to the growing popularity it gained through the literature of Burroughs, Metzner, Leary, and others in the early 1960s; and in 1976, Christian noted its involvement as a component of the healthy human brain (and perhaps as a neurotransmitter).
>
> The year 1965 marked the beginning of the use of initials, both as to substance and organisation names, in Federal Law Enforcement. It was then that, largely motivated by the psychedelic hippie movement of the younger generation at the time, the Drug Abuse Control amendments were passed and came into force. This led to the founding of the BDAC (Bureau of Drug Abuse Control), which became part of the FDA. These amendments were drafted to try to control non-narcotic substances (so-called dangerous substances) such as DMT, LSD, DET, ibogaine, bufotenine, DOM, MDA, MDMA, and TMA. BDAC was an agency that acted in parallel, but not in contact, with the already existing FBN (Federal Bureau of Narcotics), which was exclusively dedicated to the control of the three known narcotic substances: heroin, cocaine, and marijuana. . . .

32. Shulgin Alexander, Shulgin Ann. 1997. TiHKAL: the continuation. Berkeley (CA): Transform Press.

Therefore, the origin of the control of DMT as a pure substance comes from factors such as in synthesized onion, in both its pure and crystallized form, given it was synthesized even before it was discovered within countless plants, as well as to the fact that it is even found in the human brain, something that should not be so surprising given its similarity to the serotonin molecule and hence its metabolic proximity.

7.2 Ecological Reasons
A little further on, Shulgin and Shulgin (1997) continue: "The answer to the second question is that DMT is simply almost everywhere you look. It is in this flower here, in that tree there, and in those animals further away."

The book's chapter is divided into sections to indicate where DMT can be found: marine world (*S. ehina*, *S. auria*, etc.); toads (*Bufo*); herbs (birdseed or *Phalaris* species, etc.); legumes (*Acacia*, *Mimosa*, Illinois flower, *Sophora secundiflora* seed or mescal bean, etc.); *Psychotria* (*P. viridis*); limes, lemons, and Angostura bitters (*Zanthoxylum arborescens* and *Z. procerum*) (Shulgin and Shulgin 1997).

Different species of psilocybe mushrooms also grow wild around the world, as can be seen in various books. Many sources can be consulted to accredit the large number of mushrooms containing molecules that are controlled under international law (psilocin and psilocybin), but some notable ones are the following: *Psilocybin Mushrooms of the World*,[33] *Psilocibes (The Mushrooms)*,[34] *Teonanácatl*,[35] and *Pharmacotheon*.[36] Almost all varieties of psilocybin mushrooms discovered up to the time of publication can be consulted here.

---

33. Stamets P. 1996. Psilocybin mushrooms of the world: an identification guide. Berkeley (CA): Ten Speed Press.

34. Bouso JC, editor. 2013. Psilocibes: the mushrooms. Motril (Spain): Ultraradio.

35. Ott J, Bigwood J, Wasson G, Belmonte D, Hoffmann A, Weil A, Evans R. 1985. Teonanácatl: hongos alucinógenos de Europa y América del Norte [Teonanácatl (flesh of the gods): hallucinogenic mushrooms of Europe and North America]. Madrid: Swan. Spanish.

36. Ott J. 1996. Pharmacotheon. Barcelona (Spain): La Liebre de Marzo.

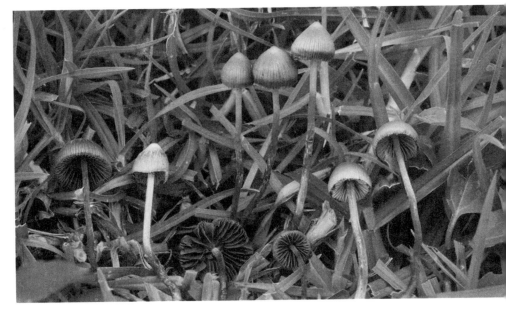

Figure 44. *Psilocybe mexicana* photographed in Veracruz, Mexico.
Image by Alan Rockefeller.

In the book *Psilocibes*, we find chapter four, authored by Oscar Parés, which lists some of the existing varieties of mushrooms that contain psilocybin: *cubensis*, *Panaeolus/Copelandia cynescens*, and *Panaeolus/Copelandia tropicalis*.

The author states:

There is a third grouping of psilocybin fungi that is worth considering. It is not distinguished from the previous two by its genetic family but by its form or presentation. Called truffle (Latin: *sclerotium*, plural: *sclerotia*), it is a hardened compact mass of mycelium containing psilocybin. It is produced when the environmental conditions are not favourable for the flower, or reproductive apparatus (read: the fungus) to sprout from the long underground mycelium. Under this heading, we would include the most widespread *Psilocybe tampanensis*, but sclerotia of *Psilocybe mexicana* and *Psilocybe atlantis* are also commercially available.

7.2.1 Psilocybe Fungi Found on the Iberian Peninsula

Following the quotation in the previous section:

> *Psilocybe cyanescens* and *Copelandia cyanescens* are also known to have been found in open fields on the Iberian Peninsula. . . .
>
> We now turn to two other psilocybe fungi of special interest that occur in the Iberian context. The first of these is *Psilocybe hispanica*. This fungus was discovered in the Huesca Pyrenees.
>
> In Galicia, we find the *Psilocybe gallaeciae*, which according to Guzmán, one of the most prestigious mycologists in the world, belongs to the variety *P. mexicana*. There are indications that two other mushrooms with psilocybin content can be found in Catalonia: *Psilocybe subbalteatus* and *Panaelus cyanescens*.

The book we have just quoted also contains a chapter titled "Visionary Fungi" in the Iberian Peninsula, written by Ignacio Seral Bozal.

To get an idea of the number of psychoactive mushrooms that are not legally controlled and exist in the Iberian Peninsula, we will cite the different sections into which this chapter is divided such as we previously did with the *TiHKAL* chapter.

- *Amanita muscaria*.[37] Species: *A. phantherina* and *A. gemmata*.
- Genus *Panaeolus*. Species: *P. cyanescens*.
- Genus *Pluteus*. Species: *P. salicinus* and *P. antricapillus*.
- Genus *Inocybe*. Species: *I. aemacta, I. corydalina, I. coelestium*, and *I. aeruginascens*.
- Genus *Gymnopilus*. Species: *G. spectabilis*.
- Genus *Psilocybe*. Species: *P. hispanicae, P. galicae, P. cyanescens*, and *P. semilanceata*.

As we can see, the argument put forward to defend the noncontrol of plants with DMT content is also applicable in the case of psilocybe

---

37. Psychoactive but not psychedelic mushroom.

mushrooms. There are many genera and species of psychoactive mushrooms in the world. Some of them, such as *A. muscaria*, do not even contain controlled molecules. Ibotenic acid and muscimol (the psychoactive ingredients of this species) are not subject to international control; therefore, in this case, it would not even raise doubts regarding varieties of mushrooms that contain controlled molecules that we are trying to resolve. Despite this lack of regulation, the consumption of this mushroom does not produce classic psychedelic effects and actually poses far more health risks than any other psilocybin-containing fungal species.

Bearing this in mind, in the case of a hypothetical control of these mushrooms, one could present the exception of the international convention that states that if the organism grows wild in that territory and there is a traditional use, reservations to the convention could be accepted.

Mescaline-containing cacti are also present not only in American countries but also in Spain and other southern European countries.

7.3 Reasons Given in the 2014 TNI Report

To understand a little more about how these international conventions were put together, let us quote a paragraph from a TNI report (Transnational Institute 2014):

> The problem regarding how to deal with the traditional uses of certain plants arose again at the 1971 Conference, especially concerning psilocybin-containing mushrooms and the mescaline-containing peyote cactus, both hallucinogenic substances listed in the 1971 Convention schedules. Then, as of now, mushrooms and peyote were used in religious and healing ceremonies by Mexican and North American Indigenous groups. Unlike the position they took during the 1961 negotiations, this time the US authorities accepted the "consensus that it is not worth trying to impose control measures on biological substances from which psychotropic substances can be obtained . . . North American Indians in the United States and Mexico use peyote in religious rites and the misuse of

this substance is considered sacrilege." By excluding plants from which alkaloids could be extracted from the scheduled lists, the 1971 Convention deviated, with good reason, from the prevailing zero-tolerance rule that had been applied in the Single Convention [on Narcotic Drugs]. The very concept of "psychotropic substances" was a distortion of the logic underpinning the control framework, as the term lacks scientific credentials and was originally invented, in effect, as an excuse to avoid the much stricter controls of the Single Convention being applied to the wide range of psychoactive, mostly synthetic, drugs included in the 1971 Convention.[38]

7.4 Conclusion

There may be several reasons as to why no plants are controlled under the 1971 Convention on Psychotropic Substances. One of the most likely reasons is the fact that if all plants containing any active substances categorized as a psychotropic were to be banned, a large part of the world's flora would be illegal. Given that in some other instances some plants are indeed controlled, it may also be that the conventions understand that it is not desirable to control plants that are not considered extremely dangerous. After all, unlike controlled plants such as the opium poppy or the coca plant, which could kill in high doses, psychedelic plant sources rarely pose a direct risk to physical health.

In conclusion, it seems that solid arguments exist such as mental health, risk and harm reduction, and what is known as the "management of risks and pleasures," and not only on a scientific but also on a historical, legal, cultural, and ecological level. These arguments can and should be taken into account by both the readers and public authorities when, with the greatest legal guarantees, facilitating access to psychedelic therapy.

---

38. Henman A, Metaal P. 2014. Hora de abrir los ojos [It's time to open our eyes]. Amsterdam (The Netherlands): Transnational Institute. Spanish.

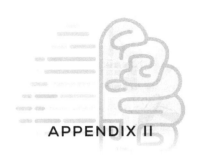

Glossary

ACTION POTENTIAL: The basic process by which communication between neurons and other cells occurs. It consists of a "shot" of electrical energy in which the concentrations of intra- and extracellular electrolytes are modified.

AGONIST: Any substance that activates a specific receptor.

ALBUMIN: Most abundant protein in the blood.

ALKALOIDS: Secondary plant metabolites, usually synthesized from amino acids, which have in common their water solubility at acidic pH and their solubility in organic solvents at alkaline pH. True alkaloids are derived from an amino acid and are therefore nitrogenous. All those with the amine or imine functional group are basic. Many psychoactive substances are alkaloids.

AMINE: Refers to endogenous amines, organic compounds derived from ammonia that constitute a large group of substances, such as serotonin or dopamine.

ANTAGONIST: Any substance that blocks the action of a given receptor.

AXON: Appendage of the neuron that can extend up to more than a meter. Its function is to send information to other cells.

BIOAVAILABILITY: The fraction of a drug or substance that ends up entering the systemic circulation and, therefore, reaching its site of action. Bioavailability is generally limited by the body's barriers when facing exogenous compounds. The more capable they are of circumventing these barriers, the greater their bioavailability.

BLOOD-BRAIN BARRIER: Complex network of blood vessels found in the brain, mainly with a very restricted permeability, precisely to protect the brain from exposure to potentially toxic substances. Although we speak of a barrier, there is no barrier as such, but rather the walls of an intricate network of vessels that could be figuratively understood as a "barrier."

BRADYCARDIA: Clinical condition in which a person has fewer than fifty heartbeats per minute. In athletes and young people, the limit of beats per minute to consider the presence of bradycardia is usually forty.

CLINICAL TEST: Any experimental study that is carried out according to certain regulations and that involves controlled exposure to certain conditions (generally drugs or molecules, but also diets, lifestyles, or any other intervention). They are carried out with healthy volunteers or patients with some disease, depending on the phase of the clinical trial in question.

CRIMINAL SIGNIFICANCE: When an alleged offense is covered by an article of the criminal code of a given state and the consequence is a legal measure consisting of a custodial sentence, a financial penalty, or the deprivation of a fundamental right, such as disqualification from holding public office, disqualification from participating in elections, or disqualification from association with the victim. There are also security measures consisting of the internment of persons who are not criminally liable, such as those who have committed the offense because of a psychiatric illness.

CYTOKINE: Protein that is synthesized by the immune system and that induces different reactions in order to defend the body against possible threats. Cytokines are mainly proinflammatory, although some of them can also be anti-inflammatory.

DAIMISTA: Parishioner of the Church of Santo Daime (ayahuasca church).

DEA: Drug Enforcement Administration. It is the agency of the U.S. Department of Justice dedicated to combating the smuggling and use of illegal drugs in the United States, as well as money laundering. Although it shares jurisdiction with the FBI, domestically, along with U.S. Immigration and Customs Enforcement and U.S. Customs and Border Protection, it is the sole agency responsible for coordinating and prosecuting antidrug investigations abroad.

DENDRITES: Extensions of the cell body. They serve the function of receiving information from their environment, mainly from other neurons.

DESIGNER DRUG: Engineering in the synthesis of new drugs whose mission is to create substances that mimic other substances under international or national control. The classic example of a designer drug would be fentanyl, which mimics controlled opiates. And the paradigm of a psychedelic designer drug would be 2CB, synthesized by A. Shulgin in 1974 in an attempt to find a molecule similar to mescaline. Terms such as NPS (new psychoactive substance) or RC (research chemicals) are also used to define these when they are very new and not yet internationally controlled.

DETOXIFICATION TREATMENT: A measure imposed by a court as a substitute for a prison sentence for drug-related offenses. The convicted person must complete the treatment under the warning that, if they fail to attend the appointments, or fail to complete the treatment, the benefit of the suspended sentence will be revoked.

DISSOCIATIVE: Can refer to substances, such as ketamine, or the effects they produce. These effects are called dissociative because they consist of a certain dissociation from body awareness. The origin of the term is attributed to Antoinette Domino, the wife of Ed Domino, an expert in psychopharmacology, who was advised by Antoinette to name ketamine and other substances "dissociatives."

EMPATHOGENIC: Category that includes substances like MDMA, due to their ability to increase empathy.

ENCEPHALON: Structure of the central nervous system that includes the cerebrum, cerebellum, and medulla oblongata.

ENDOGENOUS: Any compound or substance that is secreted naturally in our body.

ENZYMES: Proteins that produce chemical changes in all parts of the body. They help break down food, clot blood, and metabolize substances. Enzymes are found in every organ and cell in the body.

ERGOT: Popular name of the fungus *Claviceps purpurea*, an organism that colonizes cereals and is used to synthesize LSD.

EUROPEAN MONITORING CENTRE FOR DRUGS AND DRUG ADDICTION (EMCDDA): A European public agency set up to monitor and publish reports on the prevalence of drug use in the states of the European Union and to assess and advise on drug policy.

EXOGENOUS: Any compound or substance that is not found naturally in our body.

EXTRACORPOREAL EXPERIENCES: Experiences where one sees oneself outside of one's own body.

FEDERAL LAWS: Laws passed in the U.S. Congress. They differ from the laws of individual states in that they affect all American citizens and can only deal with certain very important competencies attributed by the U.S. Constitution to the U.S. Congress, located on Capitol Hill in Washington, DC. The FBI (Federal Bureau of Investigation) is responsible for investigating offenses covered by and punishable under federal law.

fMRI: Acronym for functional magnetic resonance imaging, a neuro-imaging technique. It is noninvasive and does not involve the use of radioactivity. It allows us to collect brain images while a task is being performed or while under the influence of a substance or drug.

GLUTAMATE: Essential amino acid very present in our body, closely related to the energy and activation of neurons.

HALF-LIFE: Time required for the concentrations of a drug or substance to be reduced by half. Generally, this parameter is used to calculate the time required to completely eliminate any drug or ingested substance from the body.

IATROGENIC: Harmful health consequences resulting directly from medical interventions.

ICEERS FOUNDATION: A nonprofit foundation based in the Netherlands and Spain dedicated to the research of applications of plants containing psychoactive molecules, controlled or not, for the treatment of different diseases, as well as to the protection of the cultures that use them in a traditional way. They have ECOSOC status at the United Nations Commission on Narcotic Drugs.

INTERNATIONAL CONVENTION ON PSYCHOTROPIC SUBSTANCES: Together with the 1961 Single Convention on Narcotic Drugs and the 1988 United Nations Convention against Illicit Traffic in Narcotic Drugs and Psychotropic Substances, the 1971 Convention forms the current international drug control system. It was prompted by the rise in the use of hallucinogenic or psychedelic drugs and to control nonnarcotic substances, such as those included in the 1961 Convention.

INTERNATIONAL NARCOTICS CONTROL BOARD, INCB (NCBI): An independent, quasi-judicial body of experts established under the 1961 Single Convention on Narcotic Drugs by the merger of two bodies, namely the Central Standing Committee on

Narcotic Drugs, established under the 1925 International Opium Convention, and the Narcotics Control Bureau, established under the 1931 Convention for Limiting the Manufacture and Regulating the Distribution of Narcotic Drugs. INCB consists of thirteen members, each elected to serve for a term of five years by the Economic and Social Council.

JURISPRUDENCE: Doctrine established repeatedly by the Supreme Court or the Constitutional Court, when interpreting the constitution and its laws.

LEGISLATION: A set of rules and laws that regulate the relations between people in a country or a particular sector. Legislation makes it possible to organize a given sector and a country as a whole.

LIGAND: We speak of ligands in the context of receptors and the molecules that bind to them. Any molecule that binds to a receptor can be called a ligand.

LIMBIC BRAIN: Area of the brain that contains certain structures that are highly involved in emotions and behavior. The hippocampus and the amygdala are part of the limbic brain.

LIPOPHILIC: Characteristic of substances or drugs that cause them to bind to fats (adipose tissue). The term *fat soluble* can also be used.

MAPS (MULTIDISCIPLINARY ASSOCIATION FOR PSYCHEDELIC STUDIES): A nonprofit organization founded in 1984 by Rick Doblin to research the medical and cultural uses of psychedelic substances.

METABOLISM: Set of steps through which our body processes drugs or substances. Metabolism is what allows us to more easily eliminate many of the substances or drugs that we ingest.

METABOLITE: Compound that is produced due to the metabolism of a substance. Metabolites are derivatives of the ingested molecules that are produced in the same organism. For example, when ibogaine is metabolized in the liver, noribogaine, its main metabolite, is produced.

MINISTERIAL ORDER: A legal instrument of Spanish law that is not strictly speaking a law, decree, or regulation, and which serves, in this case, to include substances in one or another list of the different national drug laws that transpose international conventions into domestic law.

MITOCHONDRIA (PLURAL OF MITOCHONDRION): Areas of the cell basically responsible for supplying energy to carry out all its functions.

MITOCHONDRIAL BIOGENESIS: Process by which the function of the mitochondria is improved. The mitochondria are structures found inside cells, closely related to the production of the energy necessary to carry out their functions properly.

MYSTICAL EXPERIENCES: Similar to peak experiences, also characterized by feelings of harmony and union, but with clearly spiritual or religious content.

NARCOTIC SUBSTANCES: These are the substances included in the 1971 Convention on Psychotropic Substances. This is a legal or juridical term that includes those substances in Schedules I and II of the 1961 Convention on Narcotic Drugs. Moreover, many of those included in this book could not be defined as narcotic drugs, but cannabis would also be defined as hallucinogenic, or semipsychedelic. And cocaine, which is not a narcotic in a strict sense, can be considered as a local anesthetic with stimulant properties.

NEOCORTEX: Most recently developed layer of the cerebral cortex, from an evolutionary point of view. It is often associated with logical thinking and most executive functions.

NEUROPLASTICITY: Flexibility of neurons expressed both functionally and anatomically. It is one of the basic characteristics of our brain.

NEUROTRANSMITTER: Chemical substance that transports, excites, and/or balances signals between neurons and cells. Some neurotransmitters are serotonin and dopamine, among many others.

NEUROTROPHIC FACTORS: Mainly BDNF and GDNF. They are proteins directly related to the induction of neuroplasticity.

PARTIAL AGONIST: Any substance that activates a certain receptor, but with a moderate or low potency, limiting its activity.

PEAK EXPERIENCES: Experiences where a person feels in complete harmony with themselves and with that which surrounds them. During these experiences there is usually a disconnection with the spatial-temporal awareness, a deep sense of well-being, and a strong sense of happiness.

PET: Acronym for positron emission tomography. This is a neuroimaging technique that requires the administration of a radioactive drug or tracer, popularly called "contrast agent." This technique records cerebral blood flow.

PHARMACODYNAMICS: Studies the effects of a drug on the body. Any physiological, biochemical, or behavioral modification is subject to pharmacodynamic analysis. It can be summed up as "what the drug does to the body."

PHARMACOKINETICS: Area of pharmacology that is dedicated to the study of the absorption, distribution, metabolism, and elimination of a drug in the body. It can be said that pharmacokinetics studies what happens to a drug from the moment it enters an organism until it is totally eliminated. It boils down to "what the body does to the drug."

PHENYLALANINE: Essential amino acid widely present in the human body. It is a precursor of adrenaline and other compounds.

PHENYLETHYLAMINES: Substances derived from phenylalanine, an essential amino acid similar to tryptophan.

PHYTOCHEMICAL PROFILE: Refers to the constituents or compounds of a given product. In the case of a plant or any natural product, its phytochemical profile will correspond to the description of the substances it contains.

PLASMA: Refers to blood plasma. It is the liquid part of the blood, mostly water rich in proteins such as albumin.

POLYPHARMACOLOGY: Paradigm developed within the field of pharmacology, especially since 2010, which consists of the use and analysis of drugs or substances with complex actions, that is to say, of those molecules or products that are not selective, acting on one or a few receptors, but are capable of modulating a large number of biological targets. This paradigm uses techniques from systems biology and has considerably advanced the knowledge of and approach to most diseases of the central nervous system, considering them as authentic systems made up of complex networks, which makes it necessary to use drugs that modulate a large number of targets that constitute these networks in order to effectively combat a given disease.

PRESUMPTIVE COLOR TEST: A field test performed by the police to provide a quick indication that a particular substance may be classified as a narcotic or psychotropic substance. It differs from confirmatory tests in that, in presumptive tests, there is a possibility of false positives and negatives, and it is not possible to quantify the purity of the substance seized and, therefore, whether it exceeds the minimum psychoactive dose, or whether it is a toxic dose. Examples of a presumptive test: Duquenois or Marquis.

PROPORTIONALITY TEST: Legal doctrine for the interpretation of conflicting fundamental rights in a legal relationship, whether these concern two fundamental rights of the individual, or a right of the individual as opposed to collective legal goods, such as public health or collective security.

PSYCHEDELIC: Can refer to a psychedelic drug or to the state that a particular psychedelic drug induces. It comes from the Greek words *psykhe* (soul, mind) and *dēlos* (manifest, reveal), meaning therefore "what reveals one's soul or mind."

PSYCHOACTIVE: A property of any substance or drug capable of modifying the state of consciousness of the user.

PSYCHOTROPIC SUBSTANCES: Those included in the 1971 Convention on Psychotropic Substances. As with narcotic drugs, this is a legal term for such substances that can be classified as stimulants (amphetamine) or hallucinogens (LSD).

REACTIVE OXYGEN SPECIES: Unstable molecules that contain oxygen and that can easily react with other molecules present in the cell, causing damage to DNA, RNA, or proteins.

RECEPTORS: Proteins or groups of proteins that are found in the cell wall and are the binding site for substances that we ingest. Receptors are one of the most common targets of many drugs or substances.

REGULATION: A rule that develops the content of a law.

RESERVATION TO AN INTERNATIONAL TREATY: A unilateral act by which a State or an international organization expresses its intention to exclude or modify an obligation arising from an international treaty.

SECOND SUMMER OF LOVE: A social phenomenon between 1988 and 1989 in the United Kingdom during which acid house music developed, providing the soundtrack for the emergence of the rave culture, a synergistic combination of a drug (namely ecstasy, where it was also known as "E") together with another way of understanding music recreationally through group dance.

SECONDARY METABOLITES: Compounds synthesized by plants and other natural products that are not essential for their survival, but are designed to satisfy their needs for interaction with the environment.

SINGLE CONVENTION ON NARCOTIC DRUGS: The international treaty signed on March 30, 1961, in New York, which forms the international legal framework for drug control. The convention defined narcotic drugs as "any of the substances in Schedules I and II, natural or synthetic," and recognizes in its preamble that the medical use of narcotic drugs is indispensable for the relief of pain and that State signatories to the treaty should take "the necessary measures to ensure the availability of narcotic drugs for such purposes."

SPECT: Acronym for single-photon emission computed tomography. It is a neuroimaging technique that requires the administration of a radioactive drug or tracer and records cerebral blood flow.

SUBCORTICAL: Refers to all the regions, neurons, or tissues of the brain that are below the cerebral cortex.

SYNAPSE: Physical connection between neurons that allows for effective communication.

SYNAPTIC CLEFT: The space between the end of one neuron and the beginning of another, and the site where the synapse is produced. The synapse is the main method of communication between neurons.

SYNERGY: Type of interaction among the components of natural products. When synergy occurs, the effect exerted is greater than the sum of the effects of all the components separately. It is important to bear in mind that this does not always take place, no matter how many components a natural product has.

SYNTHETIC: Any substance that is not extracted directly from natural products, but is the result of chemical processes and reactions carried out by human beings.

TARGET: Any site in our body where an ingested drug or substance exerts some action. Among the most common targets are receptors.

TRANSPERSONAL: Strictly speaking, it means something "that goes beyond the personal." Transpersonal psychology, for example, is a discipline that contemplates and integrates knowledge or practices of a spiritual nature, which connect the individual with realities that are greater than themselves. We talk of transpersonal experiences when we come into contact with, for example, archetypes and supposed ancestors.

TRANSPORTERS: In the context of this book and when this concept is mentioned, it refers to a heterogeneous group of proteins that collect excess neurotransmitters in the synaptic space. When there is an overexpression of transporters, neurotransmitter levels will be low, whereas when these transporters are inhibited, neurotransmitter levels will increase. The book mainly talks about serotonin (SERT) and dopamine (DAT) transporters.

TROPANE: Organic compound from which about two hundred alkaloids are derived, such as cocaine and atropine.

TROPANE ALKALOIDS: Alkaloids with a tropane nucleus, an organic compound present in different plant genera. Tropane alkaloids include atropine, scopolamine, and cocaine.

TRYPTAMINES: Molecules derived from tryptophan. Psilocybin, serotonin, and DMT are tryptamines.

TRYPTOPHAN: Essential amino acid widely present in the human body. It is the precursor to serotonin and other chemicals.

TUMOR NECROSIS FACTOR: A cytokine secreted by cells of the immune system involved in inflammatory processes and cell death. It is known by the acronym TNF.

UNIÃO DO VEGETAL (UDV): Together with Santo Daime, another of the great ayahuasca churches in the world.

UNITED NATIONS COMMISSION ON NARCOTIC DRUGS (CND): Established by the Economic and Social Council (ECOSOC) of the United Nations by Resolution 9 of February 17, 1946, as the governing body of international drug control treaties. It is a functional commission of the ECOSOC. The CND meets annually in Vienna, Austria, to examine and adopt a series of decisions and resolutions related to the implementation of drug treaties and policies about narcotic drugs and psychotropic substances.

VASOCONSTRICTION: Narrowing of the blood vessels. When blood vessels constrict, blood flow slows or is blocked. Generally, when we are cold, vasoconstriction occurs in the extremities (known as peripheral vasoconstriction) with the intention of increasing and conserving body heat in the most important areas of the body, mainly the heart.

VISUAL ANALOG SCALES (VAS): Scales commonly used in clinical practice, which consist of a 10-cm horizontal line, where the subject is asked to draw a small vertical line according to the degree to which they have experienced the phenomenon in question (such as pain, discomfort, or pleasant effects). If it is at the beginning of the line, it means they felt little or almost nothing. If more toward the end of the line, it means they felt it a lot or with a lot of intensity.

WAR ON DRUGS: A policy promoted by the U.S. government aimed at the prosecution of the production, trade, and consumption of certain psychoactive substances. The term was popularized by the media shortly after a press conference held on June 18, 1971, by then U.S. President Richard Nixon.

XENOBIOTIC: Any exogenous compound that is introduced into our body and that is not produced naturally by it.

Index

Page numbers in *italics* indicate illustrations